T0263817

Lung Transplantation

Editor

SUDISH C. MURTHY

THORACIC SURGERY CLINICS

www.thoracic.theclinics.com

Consulting Editor
M. BLAIR MARSHALL

February 2015 • Volume 25 • Number 1

ELSEVIER

1600 John F. Kennedy Boulevard • Suite 1800 • Philadelphia, Pennsylvania, 19103-2899

http://www.thoracic.theclinics.com

THORACIC SURGERY CLINICS Volume 25, Number 1
February 2015 ISSN 1547-4127, ISBN-13: 978-0-323-35452-3

Editor: John Vassallo (j.vassallo@elsevier.com)
Developmental Editor: Stephanie Carter

Thoracic Surgery Clinics (ISSN 1547-4127) is published quarterly by Elsevier Inc., 360 Park Avenue South, New York, NY 10010-1710. Months of publication are February, May, August, and November. Business and editorial offices: 1600 John F. Kennedy Boulevard, Suite 1800, Philadelphia, PA 19103-2899. Periodicals postage paid at New York, NY, and additional mailing offices. Subscription prices are $350.00 per year (US individuals), $453.00 per year (US institutions), $165.00 per year (US Students), $435.00 per year (Canadian individuals), $585.00 per year (Canadian institutions), $225.00 per year (Canadian and foreign stu-dents), $465.00 per year (foreign individuals), and $585.00 per year (foreign institutions). Foreign air speed delivery is included in all Clinics' subscription prices. All prices are subject to change without notice. **POSTMASTER:** Send address changes to Thoracic Surgery Clinics, Elsevier Health Sciences Division, Subscription Customer Service, 3251 Riverport Lane, Maryland Heights, MO 63043. **Customer Service (orders, claims, online, change of address): Telephone: 1-800-654-2452 (U.S. and Canada); 314-447-8871 (outside U.S. and Canada). Fax: 314-447-8029. E-mail: journalscustomerservice-usa@elsevier.com (for print support); journalsonlinesupport-usa@elsevier.com (for online support).**

Reprints. For copies of 100 or more, of articles in this publication, please contact Commercial Rights Department, Elsevier Inc., 360 Park Avenue South, New York, NY 10010-1710. Tel: 212-633-3874; Fax: 212-633-3820; E-mail: reprints@elsevier.com.

Thoracic Surgery Clinics is covered in *MEDLINE/PubMed (Index Medicus), EMBASE/Excerpta Medica, Science Citation Index Expanded (SciSearch®), Journal Citation Reports/Science Edition,* and *Current Contents®/Clinical Medicine.*

Contributors

CONSULTING EDITOR

M. BLAIR MARSHALL, MD, FACS
Chief, Division of Thoracic Surgery; Associate
Professor of Surgery, Department of Surgery,
Georgetown University Medical Center,
Georgetown University School of Medicine,
Washington, DC

EDITOR

SUDISH C. MURTHY, MD, PhD, FACS, FCCP
Section Head, Department of Thoracic and
Cardiovascular Surgery, Surgical Director,
Center of Major Airway Disease, Heart and
Vascular Institute, Cleveland Clinic,
Cleveland, Ohio

AUTHORS

ANDREW ARNDT, MD
Resident, Thoracic surgery, Yale New Haven
Hospital, New Haven, Connecticut

MATTHEW BACCHETTA, MD
Section of Thoracic Surgery, Price Family
Center for Comprehensive Chest Care,
Center for Acute Respiratory Care,
Columbia University Medical Center,
New York–Presbyterian Hospital, New York,
New York

MAUER BISCOTTI, MD
Section of Thoracic Surgery, Price Family
Center for Comprehensive Chest Care,
Center for Acute Respiratory Care, Columbia
University Medical Center, New York–
Presbyterian Hospital, New York, New York

DANIEL J. BOFFA, MD
Associate Professor, Thoracic Surgery, Yale
New Haven Hospital, New Heaven,
Connecticut

MARCELO CYPEL, MD, MSc
Assistant Professor, Division Thoracic Surgery,
University of Toronto, Toronto, Ontario,
Canada

R. DUANE DAVIS, MD, MBA
Professor, Director of Transplantation,
Department of Surgery, Duke University
Medical Center, Durham, North Carolina

HAYTHAM ELGHARABLY, MD
Department of Thoracic and Cardiovascular
Surgery, Cleveland Clinic, Cleveland,
Ohio

THOMAS GILDEA, MD
Department of Pulmonary, Allergy and
Critical Care Medicine, Respiratory
Institute, Cleveland Clinic, Cleveland, Ohio

BRIAN C. GULACK, MD
Department of Surgery, Duke University
Medical Center, Durham, North Carolina

MATTHEW G. HARTWIG, MD
Assistant Professor, Department of Surgery,
Duke University Medical Center, Durham,
North Carolina

DOUGLAS R. JOHNSTON, MD
Departments of Thoracic Surgery and
Cardiovascular Surgery, Heart and Vascular
Institute, Cleveland Clinic, Cleveland, Ohio

SHAF KESHAVJEE, MD, MSc, FRCSC, FACS
Director, Toronto Lung Transplant Program;
Professor, Division of Thoracic Surgery,
University of Toronto, Toronto, Ontario,
Canada

CARLI JESSICA LEHR, MD
Medical Resident, Department of Internal
Medicine, Duke University Hospital and Health
System, Durham, North Carolina

SHU S. LIN, MD, PhD
Associate Professor, Department of Surgery,
Duke University Medical Center, Durham,
North Carolina

MICHAEL MACHUZAK, MD
Department of Pulmonary, Allergy and Critical
Care Medicine, Respiratory Institute, Cleveland
Clinic, Cleveland, Ohio

DAVID P. MASON, MD
Department of Thoracic Surgery and Lung
Transplantation, Baylor University Medical
Center, Dallas, Texas

BRYAN F. MEYERS, MD, MPH
Division of Cardiothoracic Surgery,
Department of Surgery, Washington University
School of Medicine, St Louis, Missouri

JAMES M. MEZA, MD
Department of Surgery, Duke University
Medical Center, Durham, North Carolina

SUDISH C. MURTHY, MD, PhD, FACS, FCCP
Section Head, Department of Thoracic and
Cardiovascular Surgery, Surgical Director,
Center of Major Airway Disease, Heart and
Vascular Institute, Cleveland Clinic,
Cleveland, Ohio

G. ALEXANDER PATTERSON, MD
Division of Cardiothoracic Surgery,
Department of Surgery, Washington University
School of Medicine, St Louis, Missouri

GOSTA B. PETTERSSON, MD, PhD
Departments of Thoracic Surgery and
Cardiovascular Surgery, Heart and
Vascular Institute, Cleveland Clinic,
Cleveland, Ohio

VARUN PURI, MD, MSCI
Division of Cardiothoracic Surgery,
Department of Surgery, Washington
University School of Medicine, St Louis,
Missouri

JOSE F. SANTACRUZ, MD
Pulmonary, Critical Care and Sleep Medicine
Consultants, Houston Methodist, Houston,
Texas

ALEXIS E. SHAFII, MD
Department of Thoracic Surgery and Lung
Transplantation, Baylor University Medical
Center, Dallas, Texas

JOSHUA SONETT, MD
Section of Thoracic Surgery, Price Family
Center for Comprehensive Chest Care, Center
for Acute Respiratory Care, Columbia
University Medical Center, New York–
Presbyterian Hospital, New York,
New York

MARTIN STRUEBER, MD
Surgical Director, Heart and Lung
Transplantation, Heart Failure Surgery and
MCS Richard DeVos Heart and Lung
Transplant Program Spectrum Health
Hospitals, Grand Rapids, Michigan

MICHAEL Z. TONG, MD, MBA
Departments of Thoracic Surgery and
Cardiovascular Surgery, Heart and
Vascular Institute, Cleveland Clinic,
Cleveland, Ohio

DAVID WILLIAM ZAAS, MD, MBA
Associate Professor, Department of
Medicine, Duke University, Durham,
North Carolina

Contents

regards to the incidence of reflux following lung transplantation, the association of reflux with allograft dysfunction and survival, and the success of prevention and treatment of reflux in this patient population. Although antireflux surgery has been demonstrated to be safe in this population and leads to a stabilization of lung function in patients with reflux, there have not been definitive data that it improves survival.

New oxygenator technologies widened the application of extracorporeal life support significantly in the last decade. Currently the use is still limited within intensive care units. Compared to ventricular assist devices for heart failure, lung replacement technology is lagging behind, not allowing discharge on device. Challenges to achieve a true artificial lung for long term use are discussed in this article.

THORACIC SURGERY CLINICS

Preface
Lung Transplantation

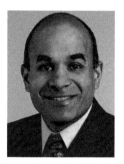

Sudish C. Murthy, MD, PhD, FACS, FCCP
Editor

Lung transplantation continues to be an imperfect science. Now, some 25 years into its run, morbidity, donor organ availability, worsening condition of candidates, and rejection all conspire to make long-term survival less than ideal. These moving parts make the orchestration of care formidable and mandate expert multidisciplinary care. Nonetheless, slow but consistent advances have been made in the field, in part attributable to many of the authors whose articles are contained herein.

Uncertainty in regard to lung transplantation begins from the very start. Selection of appropriate candidates until just less than a decade ago continued to vex clinicians. Waitlist time, once a variable in the decision-making process, has now been supplanted by the Lung Allocation Score, which represents an assessment of risk of death on a waiting list versus risk of death posttransplant. Sicker candidates are given precedence on the list, which has created some problems in deciding "how sick is too sick for transplant?" To this end, bridging strategies with extracorporeal membrane oxygenation are becoming more commonplace.

Donor organs remain in short supply, and novel approaches are being trialed to extend and expand the donor pool. Changes in the condition of the donor (postcardiac death) are being critically examined for their impact on organ quality. Ex vivo rehabilitation of organs offers the promise of salvaging unusable organs and, if validated, might double the number of donor organs. Finally, are two organs always better than one and, if not, might this serve to conserve organs and more broadly distribute them?

Postoperative care issues continue to pose challenging problems. Airway anastomotic healing issues have plagued lung transplant from the very outset and persist today. In addition to endobronchial approaches to palliate airway complications, bronchial artery revascularization is being investigated as a way to eliminate these dreaded complications altogether.

Pleural space complications can affect allograft function, and a surprising variety of insults are contributory. The gamut of complications includes nuisance pleural effusion to densely trapped lung and can dramatically impact the quality of posttransplant life. In addition, even an indolent process such as reflux may have long-reaching and intractable effects on allograft function.

Finally, as with all evolving processes, the future very quickly becomes the past, and accordingly, a brief look ahead is almost always a worthwhile undertaking. Is there a better mousetrap on the horizon? That thought is briefly explored as lung replacement theory and technology are reviewed. It is my hope that this tour through the numerous facets of lung transplantation will help focus readers' attention on current dilemmas and possible solutions and create avenues for additional thought and innovation.

Sudish C. Murthy, MD, PhD, FACS, FCCP
Section Head, Thoracic Surgery, Surgical Director
Center of Major Airway Disease
Thoracic and Cardiovascular Surgery
Cleveland Clinic
9500 Euclid Avenue, J4-1
Cleveland, OH 44195, USA

E-mail address:
murthys1@ccf.org

thoracic.theclinics.com

Thorac Surg Clin 25 (2015) ix
http://dx.doi.org/10.1016/j.thorsurg.2014.10.001
1547-4127/15/$ – see front matter © 2015 Elsevier Inc. All rights reserved.

Candidacy for Lung Transplant and Lung Allocation

Carli Jessica Lehr, MD[a],*, David William Zaas, MD, MBA[b]

KEYWORDS

- Lung transplantation • Lung allocation score • Age • Critical illness

KEY POINTS

- The Lung Allocation Score was developed in 2005 as a multi-variate model for organ allocation with the intention to decrease waiting list mortality and to allocate organs based on medical urgency.
- Diagnosis categories (Groups A-D) have been shown to impact both pre- and post-transplant survival.
- Patients over the age of 65 and critically ill patients continue to comprise a greater proportion of transplants performed each year.
- Further analysis of the outcomes following implementation of the Lung Allocation Score must continue to continue to improve patient outcomes and survival in the post-transplant period.

BACKGROUND

Lung transplantation has changed greatly since the first lung transplant was performed by J.D. Hardy in 1963 at the University of Mississippi. It took nearly 20 years for the development of cyclosporine to make transplant a viable option for patients with end-stage pulmonary disease.[1] Survival rates continued to increase through the 1980s as the number of transplants increased and cyclosporine became more widely used.[2] The growth of solid organ transplantation necessitated a national system to provide oversight over organ allocation and transplant outcomes. Congress passed the National Organ Transplant Act (NOTA) in 1984 to direct the development of a national organ transplant registry in an effort to supervise allocation processes and organ matching in the United States.[3] After the creation of NOTA, the Organ Procurement and Transplantation Network (OPTN) was created to manage allocation in conjunction with the United Network for Organ Sharing (UNOS) with the development of the Scientific Registry of Transplant Recipients (SRTR) to examine outcomes. Over the last 50 years, lung transplant outcomes have continued to improve and the lung allocation system has evolved, with a goal to maximize the net benefit provided for all donated lungs.[4,5]

Before 1995, the allocation process for lungs was solely based on wait-list time, geographic location, and blood type.[6] In 1995, a special exemption was made to allow for credit for an additional 90 days for patients with idiopathic pulmonary fibrosis (IPF) given their increased wait-list mortality; however, this did not account for variable mortality among other pulmonary diseases represented on the wait-list. The structure of the wait-list continued to select for patients able to survive for extended periods, because the time to transplant was greater than 2 years for more than half of the transplant list. Each year, the number of inactive candidates increased, to a peak of 2001 inactive candidates in 2005.[7]

The authors have nothing to disclose.
[a] Department of Internal Medicine, Duke University Hospital and Health System 2301 Erwin Road, Durham, NC 27705, USA; [b] Department of Medicine, Duke University, 2301 Erwin Road, Durham, NC 27705, USA
* Corresponding author.
E-mail address: carli.lehr@duke.edu

Thorac Surg Clin 25 (2015) 1–15
http://dx.doi.org/10.1016/j.thorsurg.2014.09.001
1547-4127/15/$ – see front matter Published by Elsevier Inc.

The structure of the wait-list led to the practice of listing patients early to provide the greatest chance to survive until transplantation and led to increased allocation for patients with more stable pulmonary disease. In response to the increasing numbers of deaths on the transplant list, the US Department of Health and Human Services instituted the Final Rule in March, 2000, which directed that medical necessity must be included in organ allocation as opposed to wait time alone.[8,9] The Lung Allocation Subcommittee was created to devise a new strategy and allocation system to comply with the mandates set forth by the Final Rule. The goals set forth by the Lung Allocation Subcommittee included reduction in mortality on the waiting list, prioritization of candidates based on clinical urgency and avoiding futile transplants, and decreasing the importance of waiting time and geography within the constraints posed by ischemic time.[10] The Lung Allocation Score (LAS) was developed as a multivariate model for allocation in an effort to decrease waiting list mortality and to alter the allocation process to provide access to organs to those patients most in need.

Numerous studies have evaluated the impact of the changing allocation methodologies on the demographics and outcomes of lung transplantation. Since 1985, the age of recipients has increased from 45 years to 55 years, and after implementation of the LAS, 10% of recipients were older than 65 years and 3% were older than 70 years.[11] Chronic obstructive pulmonary disease (COPD) was the leading indication for transplantation from 1995 to 2004, and the proportion of bilateral compared with single-lung transplants increased for every diagnosis besides cystic fibrosis (CF). Before LAS initiation, survival rates were 86% at 3 months, 76% at 1 year, 49% at 5 years, and 24% at 10 years. Survival rates continued to increase, particularly in the first 3 months after transplantation, attributable to improved operative and improved management of early posttransplant complications. In the analysis of categorical risk factors for 1-year mortality performed by the International Society for Heart and Lung Transplantation (ISHLT) in 2005, specific diseases such as primary pulmonary hypertension (PPH), IPF, and sarcoidosis were found to have greater relative risks for 1 year mortality than any identified donor/recipient or specific transplant characteristics (**Table 1**).[11] The magnitude of diagnosis continued to affect the 5-year mortality, although other continuous variables such as recipient and donor age/body mass index (BMI, calculated as weight in kilograms divided by the square of height in meters), recipient pretransplant bilirubin level, creatinine level, and pulmonary artery systolic pressure also significantly affected the risk of death.[11]

LUNG ALLOCATION SCORE

In 2004, the OPTN approved the revised LAS as a numeric score from 0 to 100 for patients aged 12 and older, which was implemented on May 4, 2005.[10] The current LAS is a numeric scoring system developed to rank patients listed for transplant both by expected transplant benefit balanced with risk of death while on the waiting list. The goal of the LAS is to prioritize objective

---

Table 1
Lung disease diagnosis group classification in the LAS

Group A	Group B	Group C	Group D
Obstructive lung disease	Eisenmenger syndrome	CF	IPF
Bronchiectasis	PPH	Immune deficiency syndromes (common variable immunodeficiency, hypogammaglobulinemia)	Sarcoidosis with mean pulmonary artery pressure >30 mm Hg
Sarcoidosis with mean pulmonary artery pressure of ≤30 mm Hg	Pulmonary vascular diseases (thromboembolic disease, veno-occlusive disease)		CREST: restrictive
Lymphangioleiomyomatosis	CREST (pulmonary hypertension)		Interstitial pneumonias
α-1-Antitrypsin deficiency	Pulmonic stenosis		Acute respiratory disease syndrome/ pneumonia
			Amyloidosis
			Connective tissue diseases Primary graft failure after lung transplant

Data from OPTN Policy 10.1.F.i. Lung disease diagnosis group classification in the Lung Allocation Score (LAS). p. 125–7.

clinical data rather than measures of clinical acuity, which can be subjective and often difficult to agree on by clinicians. A key element to the development of an equitable LAS is the comparison between survival with transplantation to survival without transplantation. Because risk of pretransplant mortality varies depending on a patient's clinical status, it is important to allow alteration of a patient's score as their clinical condition changes. Another important objective of the algorithm is the estimation of the survival benefit related to transplantation to ensure that this scarce resource would derive the greatest deal of potential benefit to patients.

Expected survival time with or without transplant in the score is calculated by measuring the area under a waiting list and 1 year posttransplant survival curves. The waiting list urgency measure is obtained by calculating the expected number of days of life without a transplant during 1 year on a wait-list. The posttransplant survival measure is defined as the expected number of days lived during 1 year after transplant. The waiting list urgency measure is subtracted from the posttransplant survival measure yielding the 1-year transplant survival benefit. It was important to provide an equal weight to both urgency and likelihood of posttransplant survival to ensure that patients in either category did not receive increased weight in the scoring system. The decision to truncate posttransplant survival at 1 year

was made based on the assumption that pretransplant factors affecting survival would have decreasing importance as time increased past 1 year (**Fig. 1**).[10]

The LAS is calculated as transplant benefit minus the waiting list urgency measure (posttransplant survival measure minus 2 times the waiting list urgency measure).[10] The LAS is calculated as a raw allocation score with values ranging between +365 to −730, which represent the 2 extremes of 100% 1-year posttransplant survival/death on waiting list and 100% waiting list 1-year survival/death on day 1 after transplant[7,12] (OPTN Policy 3.7.6.1.1). This number is normalized to a 0 to 100 scale for ease of clinical application by the formula, $100 \times$ (raw score + 2 × 365)/(3 × 365). A multitude of factors were found to be significant predictors of outcome and included in the LAS formula to determine the area under the curve, which comprises the wait-list urgency measure and posttransplant survival measure (**Tables 2–4**).

Before implementation of the LAS, the SRTR created waiting list and posttransplant models to attempt to determine hazard ratios and identify factors that affected survival. Independent risk factors were stratified into hazard models by diagnosis, and these were compared to determine if there was significant variability between alternative diagnoses.[13] Allocation scores were then compared using stratified hazards (by diagnosis) versus proportional hazards (independent risk factors) and

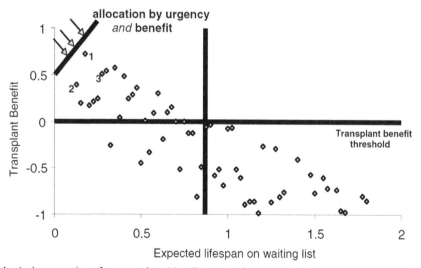

Fig. 1. Hypothetical scatterplot of expected waiting list survival versus calculated transplant benefit allocated by both benefit and urgency. Transplant benefit = expected transplant survival minus expected wait-list survival. Patients placed lower than the transplant benefit threshold experience a negative benefit from transplant. When weighting this graph equally between urgency and benefit, the angle of the best-fit line approaches 45°. The SRTR performed analyses of different angles, finding similar rates of death under 45° and increased rates of death above 60°, which resulted in adoption of the 45° model outlined earlier. (*From* Egan TM, Edwards LB, Coke MA, et al. Lung allocation in the United States. In: Lynch JP III, Ross D, editors. Lung and heart-lung transplantation (lung biology in health and disease series). New York: Marcel Dekker Inc; 2006. p. 1222; with permission; and *Data from* SRTR Analysis, 2004.)

Table 2
Equations for the calculation of the LAS

Formula	Index
$LAS = \frac{100 \times [PTAUC - 2 \times WLAUC + 730]}{1095}$ $PTAUC = \sum_{k=0}^{364} S_{TX}(k)$ $S_{TX}(t) = S_{TX,0}(t)^{exp(\alpha_1 Y_1 + \alpha_2 Y_2 + \cdots + \alpha_q Y_q)}$ $WLAUC = \sum_{k=0}^{364} S_{WL}(k)$ $S_{WL}(t) = S_{WL,0}(t)^{exp(\beta_1 X_1 + \beta_2 X_2 + \cdots + \beta_p X_p)}$	PTAUC: the area under the posttransplant survival curve (first posttransplant year) WLAUC: the area under the waiting list survival curve (in next year) β_i: coefficient for characteristics in the waiting list survival model $S_{TX}(t)$: expected posttransplant survival probability for an individual (at time t) Y_i: value of the jth characteristic for an individual candidate αRj: coefficient for characteristic j from the posttransplant model $S_{WL,0}(t)$: baseline waiting list survival probability at time t $S_{TX,0}(t)$: baseline posttransplant survival probability at time t $S_{WL}(t)$: expected waiting list survival probability for an individual candidate at time t X_i: value of the ith characteristic for an individual candidate

Data from OPTN Policy 10.1.F. The LAS calculation. p. 124.

were similar.[14] Thus, it was decided to use the proportional hazard model for increased simplicity. At the time of LAS implementation, it was determined that transplant centers were required to update clinical data used to calculate the LAS every 6 months. The only variable that may be amended less frequently is right-heart catheterization data in an effort to minimize patient risk.[7,8,14]

Since conception, the LAS has changed to incorporate both independent hazards in addition to diagnoses, because some diagnoses have independent variables that have greater severity prognostication for that particular disease. Patients are separated into 4 diagnosis groups:

obstructive lung disease (group A), pulmonary vascular disease (group B), CF/immunodeficiency disorders (group C), and restrictive lung disease (group D).[4] This grouping was created to assemble diseases by similar clinical and statistical features in an effort to provide adequate weight to diagnoses with sample sizes too small to build diagnosis-specific mortality models.[15]

ALLOCATION IN ADULTS

Lung allocation in adults is based on multiple variables, including the LAS, patient age and blood type, geography, and thoracic cavity size.

Table 3
Factors used in the waiting list mortality calculation: covariates and their coefficients

Factors Used in the Waiting List Mortality	Diagnosis Impact on Waiting List Mortality
Age	Diagnosis group B (1.57)
Bilirubin (value, increase of $\geq 50\%$)	Diagnosis group C (1.23)
BMI	Sarcoidosis with mean pulmonary artery
Cardiac index (before exercise)	pressure ≤ 30 mm Hg (0.93)
Central venous pressure (before exercise)	Bronchiectasis (0.67)
Ventilation status	Diagnosis group D (0.63)
Creatinine	Obliterative bronchiolitis (0.44)
Diabetes	Group A (0)
Diagnosis group/specific diagnoses (see **Table 1**)	Pulmonary fibrosis (−0.21)
Forced vital capacity (group D only)	Lymphangioleiomyomatosis (−0.31)
Functional status (assistance with activities of daily living)	Sarcoidosis with mean pulmonary artery pressure >30 mm Hg (−0.46)
Oxygen requirement (to maintain saturation >80%)	Eisenmenger syndrome (−0.63)
Pco_2 (≥ 40 or increase of $\geq 15\%$)	
Pulmonary artery pressure (>40 mm Hg)	
6-Minute walk distance	

Data from OPTN Policy 3.7.6.1.1. Impact factors taken from OPTN Policy 3.7.6.1.1 The LAS Calculation Table 1. p. 88–91.

Table 4
Factors used in the posttransplant survival calculation: covariates and their coefficients

Factors Used in Posttransplant Survival	Diagnosis Impact on Posttransplant Survival
Age	Eisenmenger syndrome (0.92)
Creatinine (at transplant, increase of ≥150%)	Diagnosis group B (0.62)
Cardiac index (before exercise)	Diagnosis group D (0.46)
Ventilation status	Diagnosis group C (0.36)
Oxygen requirement (to maintain saturation >80%)	Bronchiectasis (0.19)
6-Minute walk distance (if < 365 m [1200 ft])	Group A (0)
Functional status (assistance with activities of daily living)	Sarcoidosis with mean pulmonary artery pressure >30 mm Hg (−0.04)
6-Minute walk distance	Pulmonary fibrosis (−0.07)
	Sarcoidosis with mean pulmonary artery pressure ≤30 mm Hg (−0.13)
	Obliterative bronchiolitis (−1.21)
	Lymphangioleiomyomatosis (−1.52)

Data from OPTN Policy 3.7.6.1.1. Impact factors taken from OPTN Policy 3.7.6.1.1. The LAS Calculation Table 1. p. 91–3.

Geographic considerations are central to allocation to minimize organ ischemic time, leading to lung offerings first within a geographic zone. According to the OPTN Policy 3.7.10, organ allocation should first occur locally and then extend geographically through predetermined circular zones of 500, 1000, 1500, and 2500 nautical mile radii from the donor center.[12] A local zone is within the donation service area (DSA) or the organ procurement organization.

The LAS is calculated in patients aged 12 years and older and is also used for allocation of lungs from donors aged 12 years and older. For all adult donor lungs (age ≥18 years), priority first goes to recipients who are 18 years and older. In donors aged 12 to 17 years, organs are first allocated to ages 12 to 17 years, then pediatric patients (<12 years), and then, adult recipients. For donors aged 12 years and younger, lungs are first prioritized by time waiting and then priority goes first to recipients younger than 12 years, because of difficulty finding a suitable size match, then, 12 to 17 years, and then, recipients who are 18 years and older.

The allocation of organs based on age group has created many ethical concerns in patient families, the media, and those in the transplant community. Since 1985, a few adult recipients have received organs from pediatric donors (age 0–11 years), and the number of adult recipients receiving preadolescent organs has remained stable at around 10%.[11] The mortality of children on the waiting list is similar to that for adolescents and adults, although the donor pool is smaller than for older recipients.[16] Children aged 0 to 11 years are not included in the LAS system, and a high LAS does not increase their priority to receive adult lungs, although the use of partial lobar transplants had been successful in pediatric patients. In this situation, the organs are offered to all acceptable candidates aged 12 years and older in the region. This protocol has prompted practice-changing legislation, allowing patients like Sarah Murnaghan and Javier Acosta, pediatric patients with end-stage CF, to be considered for listing on the adult lung transplant list on a case-by-case basis with the OPTN review board. These recent changes in legislation allow select patients younger than the age of 12 years to be considered for evaluation by LAS and allow for eligibility for adult lungs or lobar transplants based on their disease severity. In addition, it has been proposed that the donor pool be expanded by changing legislation to increase priority for access to adolescent donors to pediatric recipients.[16,17]

ALLOCATION IN ADOLESCENTS (AGES 12–17 YEARS)

Allocation in adolescents (aged 12–17 years) is similar to that in the adult population, with the exception that available donor organs are first offered to adolescent candidates. Further allocation is similar to adults, with geographic preference first to local candidates who are ABO identical and then to local candidates who are ABO compatible. If no candidates are identified, preference then goes to child recipients (<12 years). Donor lungs are offered to local adult candidates only if there are no suitable local adolescent or child recipients. The recipient range is then expanded to the same zones, A, B, C, D, and E, as are used in adult organ allocation.[4,12]

ALLOCATION IN CHILDREN YOUNGER THAN 12 YEARS

Children are grouped together from ages 0 to 11 years in the lung allocation schema, and transplantation is not governed by the LAS. At the time of LAS development, children were not included, because the impact of diagnoses had the potential to make the LAS a poor prognostic indicator for severity of disease and required transplant urgency. Children are designated as either priority 1 or priority 2, depending on meeting a specific set of predetermined criteria. To become priority 1 status, a candidate must have 1 or more of the following: respiratory failure, pulmonary hypertension, or an exception case reviewed by the Lung Review Board[12] (OPTN Policy 3.7.6.2) (**Box 1**).

Preference is given to patients in priority 1 based on ABO compatibility followed by contiguous time spent as priority 1 status. Multiple episodes of priority 1 status cannot be combined to increase waiting time, although it is contributory in situations in which there is a tie between priority 1 candidates. Ties are determined based on total waiting time, which is defined as the summation of time spent as priority 1, priority 2, and inactive time[12] (OPTN Policy 3.7.9.3). The ranking of priority 2 candidates is determined by total waiting time, and clinical data must be updated every 6 months to maintain priority 1 status on the waiting list. Candidates maintain their priority 2 status if they are identified as requiring an organ by their transplant center.

Donor organs in children younger than 12 years first are allocated to ABO identical priority 1 pediatric recipients within the local DSA, zone A, and zone B combined. If no recipients are found, then, priority 1 ABO compatible donors from the same geographic area are selected, followed by priority 2 candidates. Donor lungs are then offered successively to adolescent ABO identical candidates from DSA and zone A, adult ABO identical candidates from DSA and zone A, adult ABO compatible candidates from DSA and zone A. If no suitable candidates are identified in the DSA and zone A, priority then moves to adolescents in zone B, then, adults in zone B, and then, to children in zone C. If there are still no suitable matches, the net is cast wider to include first adolescents in zone C, followed by adults in zone C, and to zones D and E[4,12] (OPTN Policy 3.7.11).

CHANGES TO THE LUNG ALLOCATION SCORE SINCE CONCEPTION

The first alteration to the LAS came in 2008, when the P_{CO_2} value was incorporated into the LAS calculation after analysis indicating that P_{CO_2} values affected wait-list mortality and posttransplant survival outcomes.[18] The LAS incorporates both current P_{CO_2} and change in P_{CO_2} measured by the threshold change ([highest P_{CO_2}–lowest P_{CO_2}]/lowest P_{CO_2}) and threshold change maintenance ([current P_{CO_2}–lowest P_{CO_2}]/lowest P_{CO_2}). The threshold change evaluates if the change in P_{CO_2} is greater than 15% and the threshold change maintenance is an additional value that the candidate receives after the impact from the threshold change. This value determines the candidate's ability to benefit from the impact given to the LAS from the threshold change[12] (OPTN Policy 3.7.6.1.3).

The addition of bilirubin to the LAS also came in 2008, although the logistics of implementation have progressed slowly. Bilirubin measurements make little difference for most transplant candidates but have a high impact factor for some candidates with idiopathic pulmonary hypertension (group B). In group B patients, an increase in bilirubin level of greater than 50% from time of listing increases risk of death while on the waiting list.[19] As in P_{CO_2} measurements, bilirubin levels are measured by current bilirubin and change in bilirubin, which is accounted for by 2 change

---

Box 1
Determination of priority 1 child candidates

Candidates must have one of the following:

- Respiratory failure
  - Requiring continuous mechanical ventilation or
  - Requiring supplemental oxygen to sustain F_{IO_2} greater than 50% to maintain oxygen saturation levels greater than 90% or
  - Arterial/capillary P_{CO_2} greater than 50 mm Hg, or a venous P_{CO_2} greater than 56 mm Hg
- Pulmonary hypertension
  - Stenosis of pulmonary veins involving 3 or more vessels
  - Showing suprasystemic pulmonary artery pressure on cardiac catheterization or echocardiogram
  - Cardiac index less than 2 L/min/m^2
  - Syncope
  - Hemoptysis

Data from OPTN Policy 3.7.6.2. Candidates Aged 0–11. p. 106–7.

calculations: threshold change ([highest bilirubin–lowest bilirubin]/lowest bilirubin) and threshold change maintenance ([current bilirubin–lowest bilirubin]/lowest bilirubin).

Additional changes include the removal of forced vital capacity (FVC) in all groups except group D diagnoses, because this did not have statistical significance in the revised waiting list model. There have also been minor changes related to the weighting of factors within the model. The last changes made to the LAS were in 2012, and further changes are anticipated as more factors affecting mortality are studied and tested within the current model.[20] In addition, as data continues to be analyzed through large-scale descriptive studies such as REVEAL registry (Registry to Evaluate Early and Long-term Pulmonary Arterial Hypertension Disease Management) and the Lung Retrospective Data Collection Projects, it is expected that more data will become available to continue to adapt the model as the characteristics of patients on the waiting list continue to evolve.[20,21]

PRIMARY DIAGNOSIS AND EFFECT ON LUNG ALLOCATION SCORE

Patients on the waiting list had vastly different survival times, and the implications of diagnosis on wait-list mortality were thoroughly investigated before implementation of the LAS. The 4 primary diagnoses taken into consideration include COPD, idiopathic pulmonary arterial hypertension (IPAH), CF, and IPF. Based on data in the OPTN/SRTR database from 2001 to 2002, mortality on the wait-list was 9.7%, 13.1%, 17.8%, and 23.1% for group A, B, C, and D diagnostic groups, respectively.[13] Each of these diseases has different risk factors associated with increased patient mortality. Patients with low wait-list mortality, such as those with COPD, had a greater chance of survival to transplantation with the system before the LAS. Development of the LAS greatly affected the impact of diagnostic grouping on likelihood of transplant (**Fig. 2**).

GROUP A: CHRONIC OBSTRUCTIVE PULMONARY DISEASE

COPD accounted for a total of 14,784 lung transplants from January, 1995 to June, 2012. Before the implementation of the LAS, COPD (both A1ATD [Alpha-1 anti-trypsin deficiency] and non-A1ATD) represented most lung transplants performed. COPD comprised 35.4% of transplants from 1990 to 2004, with a decrease to 30.9% of transplants after 2005, although non-A1ATD COPD decreased from 40% to 30%.[13] The pre-LAS allocation system led to increased transplant in patients with COPD given their high survival rates at 80% and 70% at 2 and 3 years after listing.[22]

In patients with COPD, factors contributing to waiting list mortality included hospitalization, steroid dependency, FEV_1, O_2 requirement at rest, BMI, and age.[8,10,13,23] The factors contributing to the 1-year posttransplant mortality included hospitalization at time of transplant, age, and center

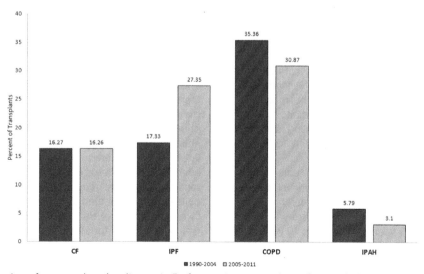

Fig. 2. Indications for transplant by diagnosis (before LAS compared to after LAS). (*Adapted from* Yusen RD, Christie JD, Edwards LB, ISHLT. The Registry of the International Society for Heart and Lung Transplantation: thirtieth adult lung and heart-lung transplant report–2013; Focus theme: age. J Heart Lung Transplant 2013;32(10):965–78; with permission.)

volume.[8,10,13] In a study published in the *American Journal of Transplantation* in 2009 by Titman and colleagues,[22] a survival benefit was identified in patients with COPD, although it was less than in other diagnostic groupings, which was also supported by 2 earlier European studies.[24,25] Median survival is 5.4 years and average conditional median survival for patients surviving to 1 year after transplantation is 6.9 years in non-A1ATD and 8.7 years in those with ATATD-related COPD. Patients with COPD have the lowest unadjusted 3-month mortality, of 9% after transplantation.[7,13] However, the implementation of the LAS had a significant impact on the indications for transplant. The percentage of patients with COPD continues to decline slowly after implementation of the LAS, and IPF has surpassed COPD as the most prevalent transplant diagnosis.

GROUP B: IDIOPATHIC PULMONARY HYPERTENSION

Based on data compiled in the REVEAL registry, for patients enrolled between 2006 and 2009, the 1-year, 3-year, and 5-year survival in patients with pulmonary arterial hypertension were 85%, 68%, and 57%.[26,27] The cause of death in most patients is progressive right-sided heart failure and combined heart-lung transplant (HLT) and double-lung transplant has been associated with improved long-term outcomes when compared with single-lung transplant in IPAH.[28] IPAH has accounted for a total of 1160 lung transplants since 1995.[7] Factors contributing to waiting list mortality in this group include hospitalization, mechanical ventilation, steroid dependency, and wedge pressure, with risk factors for posttransplant mortality of intensive care unit (ICU) status, single-lung transplant, and increased BMI.[7,10,23]

Group B patients make up 5.1% of the waiting list, a decrease from 8.3%, and the average wait time is 9.7 months.[7] Based on the most recent ISHLT data from 2013, the median survival of patients with IPAH with lung transplant is 5.2 years, with a conditional median survival for patients surviving the first year of 10.0 years.[13,28] Patients with IPAH made up 23% of HLT recipients from June, 2000 to June, 2012 and survival after HLT has improved, particularly in the early posttransplant period. Survival for all-comers was 63% at 1 year, 44% at 5 years, and 31% at 10 years; however, patients who survived the first year after HLT had a median survival of 3.3 years and a conditional median survival of 10 years, which did not differ among pretransplant diagnoses.[11] A retrospective study performed by Schaffer and colleagues[29] comparing lung transplantation in the pre-LAS and post-LAS eras found a statistically significant increase in the incidence of transplantation as well as decreased wait-list mortality in patients with IPAH in the post-LAS era.[11] An additional study performed by Chen and colleagues[30] found an increased likelihood of transplantation and an unchanged wait-list mortality, without a change in posttransplant mortality.

Higher cardiac index is an independent predictor for improvement in survival in patients with IPAH and is an important component to the LAS in this patient population.[28] The addition of bilirubin to the LAS also benefits patients with IPAH, because this can be a surrogate marker for hepatic congestion caused by worsening right-heart function. Although the number of patients listed on the waiting list who went to transplant increased after implementation of the LAS, IPAH represented a decreased percentage of all organ recipients (5.8% before the LAS, and 3.2% after LAS), raising the concern that the LAS may not adequately assign priority to this patient population.[28,30] As of 2011, group B candidates made up 5.1% of the waiting list and have a median wait time of 9.7 months.[7] Patients with IPAH also have the highest unadjusted 3-month mortality at 22%, although average survival after transplantation is 10 years.[11]

The implementation in the LAS coincided with increasing use of improved end-stage pulmonary hypertension therapies, such as inhaled iloprost and oral sildenafil. Sildenafil was approved by the US Food and Drug Administration for use in pulmonary hypertension in 2005 after it was studied in multiple trials showing improvement in World Health Organization functional class, exercise capacity, and hemodynamics.[31–33] In addition, inhaled iloprost was approved in 2004 for severe pulmonary hypertension.[33,34] It is difficult to ascertain whether improved wait-list survival and decreased transplantation is caused by LAS implementation or by improved pharmacologic therapies. Since that time, additional therapies in the categories of prostacyclin analogues, phosphodiesterase 5 inhibitors, endothelin receptor antagonists, and soluble guanylate cyclase stimulators have entered the market, significantly affecting the treatment of severe pulmonary hypertension. The most recent study by Schaffer and colleagues[29] indicated a dramatic improvement in the incidence of transplantation, with reduced wait-list mortality for end-stage patients, many of whom are refractory to advanced medical therapies. In addition, these investigators found a survival advantage associated with listing at medium-volume to high-volume centers that was postulated to be caused by access to advanced IPAH therapies.

GROUP C: CYSTIC FIBROSIS

The 2013 report of the ISHLT indicates that patients with CF make up the third largest diagnosis group undergoing transplant: 16.3% of all lung transplants performed in the last 15 years, with a median survival of 7.8 years, with a conditional median survival of 10.5 years.[11,35,36] Predictors for waiting list mortality include hospitalization, steroid dependency, diabetes, wedge pressure, FVC % predicted, cardiac output, and BMI, with posttransplant mortality risk factors of drug-related peptic ulcer disease before listing.[7,10,23]

Adoption of the LAS did not change the percentage of transplants for CF. Thabut and colleagues[37] performed a study published in 2013 evaluating survival benefit of lung transplant for patients with CF after the implementation of the LAS. In their study cohort of 704 adult patients with CF, they found that 39.3% received a transplant at 3 months, 64.7% at 12 months, with death rates while on the wait list of 8.5% and 12.9%, respectively. Survival after transplant was 96.5% at 3 months, 88.4% at 12 months, and 67.8% at 3 years. The investigators found that lung transplant decreased the risk of death by 69% in their cohort. This study used the LAS as a proxy for patient severity on the waiting list and found that a higher LAS was associated with a statistically significant increase in survival benefit for lung transplant.[37] Before this study, 9 studies assessed the survival benefit of lung transplant in patients with CF, with mixed results.[35]

GROUP D: IDIOPATHIC PULMONARY FIBROSIS

Lung transplant has been shown to improve both survival and quality of life in patients with severe interstitial lung disease (ILD) that is refractory to medical therapy.[38] After transplantation for IPF, patients have a median survival of 4.5 years, with a conditional median survival of 7 years, similar to group A and B diagnoses.[11] The survival time may in addition be affected by the increased age of diagnosis compared with patients with CF. Historically, patients with IPF have been poor candidates for transplant, given their advanced age and multiple comorbidities. Before the implementation of the LAS, patients with IPF experienced the highest death rate while on the waiting list for transplantation when compared with CF and COPD.[8,39] Risk factors for waiting list mortality in patients with IPF include hospitalization, mechanical ventilation, steroid dependency, and wedge pressure, with posttransplant mortality risk factors including ICU status, single-lung transplant, and higher BMI.[7,10,23] As IPF progresses, the development of pulmonary hypertension significantly increases the risk for posttransplant pulmonary complications and decreased survival.[40]

A study performed by De Oliveira and colleagues[41] showed that patients with IPF after 2005 had a higher LAS of 43.3 compared with those before 2005, with an average LAS of 38.3 without increased rates of postoperative mortality, and also noted that the waiting list time decreased from 266 days before LAS to a mere 78 days in the post-LAS transplant model. The investigators also found that patients in the post-LAS era are not only transplanted more frequently, representing 27.4% of transplants compared with 17.3%, but also are older, require increasing amounts of supplemental oxygen before transplant, and have lower cardiac indices.[41] After the advent of the LAS, patients with IPF made up 12% of waiting list recipients, a 6% decrease from the previous year, representative of the increase in IPF transplants to 28% from 24% in just 1 year.[39] In the most recently published 2011 OPTN/SRTR Annual Data Report, group D made up 46.1% of waiting list candidates, with a median waiting time of only 2.1 months.[7] Although patients with IPF make up a significant number of lung transplant recipients, they have documented decreased posttransplant survival, particularly in the early posttransplant period, compared with other indications for lung transplant.[42]

AGE IN TRANSPLANT

There are many transplant centers that continue to use an age cutoff of 65 years for transplant eligibility, because advanced age in transplant recipients has been identified as a risk factor for increased posttransplant mortality.[13] Patients older than 55 years begin to experience an increased 1-year mortality, which increases with age. However, patients older than 65 years have similar rates of diabetes, hypertension, acute rejection, and renal dysfunction compared with younger patients, although they experience an increased incidence of skin cancers.[11] Many proponents of increasing eligibility for older recipients dispute the validity of chronologic age compared with the importance of functional age in posttransplant outcomes. After implementation of the LAS in 2005, the subgroup of recipients aged 65 years and older have increased most rapidly.[43] Patients aged 65 and older comprised less than 5% of transplant recipients in 2002 and increased to 19% in 2008 and 26.6% in 2011.[7,11,44]

A consensus report published by the ISHLT in 2006[45] recommended that age older than 65 years should serve as a relative contraindication to lung transplant based on registry data indicating reduced survival in this age cohort. The ISHLT 30th Adult Lung and Heart-Lung Transplant report indicated a median survival of 3.6 years in patients older than 65 years, compared with 6.5 years in those aged 35 to 49 years, with a 5-year survival of 38% for patients older than 65 years, 46% for those 60 to 65 years, and 52% to 57% for patients younger than age 60 years.[11] Two studies published after implementation of the LAS reported no difference in both 1-year and 3-year survival rates compared with younger patient cohorts.[46,47]

A retrospective cohort study was performed by Genao and colleagues[43] evaluating 4805 patients who received a lung transplant between 2005 and 2009, stratifying patients by age 65 years or older compared with those younger than 65 years. Functional status was measured by Karnofsky performance score (KPS) before and after transplantation, and investigators found that older age was not associated with different rates of decline in KPS over time and that the rate of functional decline was not greater in patients aged 70 years and older compared with age 65 to 69 years. A recent study performed by Kilic and colleagues[48] evaluated the outcomes of lung transplantation in patients older than 70 years after implementation of the LAS in 2005 and found that outcomes in patients 70 years and older are comparable with outcomes in those aged 65 to 69 years. The most recently published OPTN/SRTR Annual Data Report from 2011 indicates that candidates older than 65 years continue to be added faster than any other age group and comprise 24.4% of the waiting list, a stark change from a mere 2.9% of candidates in 1998 (**Fig. 3**).[7]

DISPARITIES IN TRANSPLANT

Racial disparities in lung transplantation have improved with the introduction of the LAS, although gender disparities have increased.[49] Wille and colleagues[49] performed a study of 8806 registered waiting list patients and found that black patients were less likely to undergo transplantation before LAS compared with white recipients (56.3% vs 69.2%; odds ratio [OR] 0.54; $P<.001$), which improved in the LAS era (86% vs 87%; OR 1.07, $P = .74$). The percentage of female lung transplants also decreased to 41.9% in 2011 compared with 53.5% in 2001, which may be caused by a decreased number of female donors.[7] Women had an increased likelihood of death or critical illness precluding transplant compared with men after implementation of the LAS (16.1% vs 11.3%; OR 1.58, $P<.001$) compared with the pre-LAS system (33.4% vs 30.7%; OR 1.19, $P = .08$).[49] To our knowledge, no studies have been performed that address other racial or ethnic groups that aid in the understanding of unintended consequences caused by the LAS system.

Given the focus of geographic regions in the LAS, it is important to consider the potential for geographic disparities when comparing the pre-LAS and post-LAS eras. Before implementation of the LAS, listing and lung transplantation was shown to be reduced for patients living in rural areas without a transplant center in close proximity.[50] A study performed by Thabut and colleagues[50] indicated that the LAS did not diminish

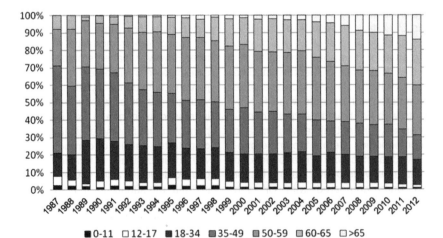

■ 0-11 □ 12-17 ■ 18-34 ■ 35-49 ▨ 50-59 ▨ 60-65 □ >65

Fig. 3. Age in transplant. (*Adapted from* Yusen RD, Christie JD, Edwards LB, ISHLT. The Registry of the International Society for Heart and Lung Transplantation: thirtieth adult lung and heart-lung transplant report–2013; Focus theme: age. J Heart Lung Transplant 2013;32(10):965–78; with permission.)

these geographic disparities. However, this study did not identify decreased transplantation rates or clinical follow-up once patients were listed. This study was unable to identify if these disparities were caused by reduced rural referral rates, reduced listing, or personal preference of patients in these remote locations. Furthermore, improvements to the current allocation system to mitigate geographic disparities in transplant listing will be an important consideration as further modifications are made to the LAS.

CRITICAL ILLNESS BEFORE TRANSPLANT

Before the development of the LAS in 2005, critically ill patients were at a significant disadvantage, because the primary determinant for transplant was time spent on the waiting list.[51] Critically ill patients have historically contributed to approximately 10% of deaths on the waiting list. Although the LAS model incorporates both the risk of 1-year wait-list mortality and 1-year posttransplant survival, wait-list mortality carries a greater weight in the algorithm.[10] There has been debate after implementation of the LAS as to the effect of the score on survival as well ass studies showing increased ICU time and greater rates of primary graft dysfunction.[52] A study was performed by Russo and colleagues[53] to address the association between the LAS at time of transplantation and postoperative morbidity and mortality. This study grouped 3386 patients into LAS of less than 50 (n = 3161), LAS 50 to 75 (n = 411), and LAS greater than 75 (n = 197), with a primary outcome of posttransplant graft survival at 1 year and secondary outcomes of in-hospital complications and length of stay. The study found that LAS greater than 75 was associated with significantly decreased survival in the first year (proportion alive 0.82 in LAS >75 compared with 0.89–0.93 in LAS <75) and increased complications during the transplant hospitalization; however, there was no difference between LAS in the incidence rate of death during years 1 to 3 after transplant.[53] The rate of change in LAS is also critical to posttransplant survival, and a study from Tsuang and colleagues[54] reported that 702 patients with a change in LAS greater than 5 had a significantly worse posttransplant survival (hazard ratio 1.31; 95% CI 1.11–1.54), even when adjusted for LAS at time of transplantation. In patients with an LAS greater than 50, a program must update the status of assisted ventilation, supplemental oxygen, and current Pco_2 every 14 days to ensure the most accurate clinical data.[20]

Historically, extracorporeal membrane oxygenation (ECMO) as a bridging strategy to lung transplantation has been associated with poor outcomes.[55–57] As technology continues to improve, outcomes continue to improve as ECMO patients are becoming ambulatory and managed with minimal sedation.[58,59] A recent study performed by Fuehner and colleagues[60] compared 26 patients bridged to lung transplant with 34 historical control patients receiving invasive mechanical ventilation with a significant survival advantage in the awake ECMO group, of 80% versus 50%. A study performed by Turner and colleagues[58] focusing on incorporation of rehabilitation and physical therapy in 3 patients awaiting transplantation on ECMO reported positive posttransplant outcomes, with all patients being weaned from the ventilator and becoming ambulatory within 1 week after transplant. Although ECMO is not yet the standard of care before transplantation, it provides a valuable strategy for patients who would otherwise be unable to survive to transplant. These patients have survival that is comparable with and often improved compared with traditional mechanical ventilation, with further improvement expected as awake and ambulatory ECMO begin to emerge as standards of care in ECMO bridging protocols.

Malnutrition in critically ill patients significantly increases posttransplant morbidity and mortality. In a study of 453 patients undergoing lung transplantation, performed by Chamogeorgakis and colleagues,[61] 9% to 25% of patients carried a diagnosis of malnutrition defined by a BMI less than 18.5, weight/height ratio 0.3 or less, albumin less than 3.5 g/dL, total protein less than 6 g/dL, and an absolute lymphocyte count less than 1000. In this study, the investigators found that hypoalbuminemia (<3 g/dL) was associated with increased 1 year posttransplant mortality.[61] A UNOS study performed by Allen and colleagues[62] assessed the effect of BMI on posttransplant outcomes in 11,411 patients, with evidence of increased risk of death with patients who are both under weight and over weight.

CURRENT IMPLICATIONS AND FURTHER DIRECTIONS FOR ALLOCATION

In the years after the LAS, the number of transplants continues to increase, with 1830 lung transplants performed in 2011, 70.1% bilateral and 29.9% single-lung transplants, and 3.8% retransplants. The wait-list number continues to increase, with 2200 new candidates added to the list in 2011, and donation rates have been unable to match the increasing demand. Donation rates have continued to increase over the past 10 years, with the largest contribution from donors aged 15 to 34 years, with an increase from 7.4 to 13.7

donations per 100 deaths over the past 10 years.[7] The decrease in inactive candidates on the waiting list since implementation of the LAS suggests that patients are being listed at an optimal time and that the transplant process may be occurring more efficiently. The proportion of patients who receive a lung transplant within 1 year of listing is on average 64.4%, although this varies significantly based on the DSA.[7]

The median LAS at transplantation continues to increase: 40.8 in 2011 with 6.3% of wait-listed patients with an LAS of greater than 50 compared with 36.6 in 2005 with less than 2% of wait-listed patients with an LAS greater than 50. A critical issue in the current algorithm is the increased weight given to pretransplant mortality, which may promote allocation of scarce organs to patients with low posttransplant mortality. In the study by Russo and colleagues,[53] patients with LAS from 90 to 100 and 80 to 90 had an expected survival of only 1.56 and 2.28 years, respectively. According to the most recent OPTN/SRTR 2011 annual report, the incidence of primary graft failure decreased to 5.3% and decreased long-term graft failure. This report delineated a clear relationship between worsening LAS and decreased graft survival.[7]

These findings have led many to suggest the possibility for alternative transplantation strategies for patients with extremely high scores. For example, in heart transplantation, risk of posttransplant mortality higher than a defined level leads to reduction of transplantation priority or placement on an alternative transplant list.[63] This strategy could permit high-risk recipients to receive only organs that are not suitable for standard recipients in an effort to extract the greatest benefit from the scarce resource of donated organs. Further study is needed regarding addition of other prognostic factors in the 4 diagnostic groupings to provide the most equitable ranking system based on disease-specific markers of clinical severity.

Results of studies analyzing posttransplant survival after LAS are conflicting, with a study performed by Kozower and colleagues[52] from 2008 identifying increased incidence of primary graft dysfunction and longer ICU stay in the post-LAS era, although there was similar 1-year survival. A study performed by McCue and colleagues[64] found no difference in posttransplant morbidity and a small, although statistically significant, 1-year survival advantage in the post-LAS era. A review article by Hachem and colleagues[65] presented data from UNOS indicating a largely unchanged survival rate, with a 2-year survival of 72.23% in patients transplanted between 2000

and 2005 compared with a 2-year survival of 70.14% in patients transplanted between 2005 and 2006.[7] Promising data in the most recent publication by ISHLT in 2013 indicate that from 1988 to 2011, the 1-year survival improved from 70% (1988–1994) to 81% (2004–2011). In a Kaplan-Meier survival analysis performed by ISHLT in 2005 for transplants performed between 1994 and 2003, mean survival was 4.8 years for COPD, PPH 4.3 years, CF 5.8 years, and IPF 3.7 years. This finding can be compared with ISHLT Kaplan-Meier survival analysis from 2013[11] documenting patients with transplants performed between 1990 and 2011 with 5.4 years for COPD, IPAH 5.2 years, CF 7.6 years, and ILD 4.5 years.

Wait-list times have continued to decrease since 2005 for diagnosis groups B, C, and D (9.7, 3.7, and 2.1 months, respectively), with an unchanged time to transplant in group A (7.0 months). In 2004, transplant rates per 100 patient years on the waiting list for group A, B, C, and D were 34.1, 7.0, 35.5, and 34.8, respectively, whereas in 2011, these increased across all groups, with rates in group A, B, C, and D of 66.3, 46.9, 119.5, and 165.9, respectively. Mortality in the first year after transplant continues to improve with each passing year, and in 2011, 1-year mortality was 14%, a significant decrease from 23% in 2001. Initially, waiting list mortality improved after the implementation of the LAS, but these are increasing, with a mortality of 15.7 per 100 wait-list years, which may be a reflection of transplantation of critically ill patients with increasing age representation in the waiting list population.[7]

The LAS fundamentally changed the landscape of lung transplant. The main goals of LAS implementation were to decrease wait-list mortality, decrease waiting time, and improve posttransplant survival rates. Although it is yet to be seen what the long-term sequelae are from this change, reports indicate that survival after transplantation continues to improve for each disease class and that both critically ill and older patients are receiving transplants more frequently. The LAS will continue to evolve as additional data arise regarding disease-specific parameters that are predictive for better and worse outcomes.

REFERENCES

1. Morris PJ. The impact of cyclosporin A on transplantation. Adv Surg 1984;17:99–127.
2. Cooper JD, Pearson FG, Patterson GA, et al. Technique of successful lung transplantation in humans. J Thorac Cardiovasc Surg 1987;93(2):173–81.
3. Gore A, Hatch O. National Organ Transplant Act of 1984. In: Senate 2048–98th Congress: Sec. 101-

Sec, vol. 401. Washington, DC: 1984. p. 98–507. Weekly Compilation of Presidential Documents, Presidential statement. Available at: http://history.nih.gov/research/downloads/PL98-507.pdf. Accessed October 7, 2014.

4. Colvin-Adams M, Valapour M, Hertz M, et al. Lung and heart allocation in the United States. Am J Transplant 2012;12(12):3213–34.

5. UNOS. Fact sheets: timeline of key events in US transplantation and UNOS history. 2013. Available at: http://www.unos.org/donation/index.php?topic=history. Accessed January 29, 2014.

6. OPTN/SRTR. OPTN/SRTR 1990 Annual Report of the US Scientific Registry for transplant recipients and the Organ Procurement and Transplantation Network-transplant data: 1988–1991. Richmond (VA); Bethesda (MD): UNOS and the Division of Organ Transplantation; Bureau of Health Resources Development; Health Resources and Services Administration; US Department of Health and Human Services; 1990.

7. Valapour M, Paulson K, Smith JM, et al. OPTN/SRTR 2011 annual data report: lung. Am J Transplant 2013;13(Suppl 1):149–77.

8. OPTN/SRTR. OPTN/SRTR, 2005, 2009 Annual reports of the US organ procurement and transplantation network and the scientific registry of transplant. recipients: transplant data 1999–2008. Bethesda (MD): Health Resources and Services Administration, US Department of Health and Human Services; 2009.

9. Department of Health and Human Services. Final rule, 42 CFR 121: Organ procurement and transplantation network. Federal Register 42 CFR (Part 121). 1999. p. 56649–61. Available at: http://www.gaonet.gov/special.pubs/organ/appendd.pdf. Accessed October 7, 2014.

10. Egan TM, Murray S, Bustami RT, et al. Development of the new lung allocation system in the United States. Am J Transplant 2006;6(5 Pt 2):1212–27.

11. Yusen RD, Christie JD, Edwards LB, et al. The registry of the international society for heart and lung transplantation: thirtieth adult lung and heart-lung transplant report-2013; focus theme: age. J Heart Lung Transplant 2013;32(10):965–78.

12. Organ Procurement and Transplantation Network. Policy 10 (Previously 3.7.6). Allocation of thoracic organs. Available at: http://optn.transplant.hrsa.gov/ContentDocuments/OPTN_Policies.pdf#named-dest=Policy_10. Accessed October 7, 2014.

13. Christie JD, Edwards LB, Kucheryavaya AY, et al. The Registry of the International Society for Heart and Lung Transplantation: twenty-eighth adult lung and heart-lung transplant report—2011. J Heart Lung Transplant 2011;30(10):1104–22.

14. Egan TM, Edwards LB, Coke MA, et al. Lung allocation in the United States. In: Lynch JP III, Ross D, editors. Lung and heart-lung transplantation (lung biology in health and disease series). New York: Marcel Dekker; 2006. p. 490–5.

15. Egan T, Bennett LE, Garrity ER, et al. Are there predictors of death at the time of listing for lung transplant? J Heart Lung Transplant 2002;21(1):154.

16. Snyder JJ, Salkowski N, Skeans M, et al. The equitable allocation of deceased donor lungs for transplant in children in the United States. Am J Transplant 2014;14(1):178–83.

17. Sweet SC, Barr ML. Pediatric lung allocation: the rest of the story. Am J Transplant 2014;14(1):11–2.

18. OPTN. Implementation of addition of current and change in PCO2 to the lung allocation calculation in UNetSM. Richmond (VA): United Network for Organ Sharing; 2008.

19. Kramer M, Marshall SE, Tiroke A, et al. Clinical significance of hyperbilirubinemia in patients with pulmonary hypertension undergoing heart-lung transplantation. J Heart Lung Transplant 1991;10(2):317.

20. OPTN. Proposal to revise the lung allocation score (LAS) system. 2013. Available at: http://optn.transplant.hrsa.gov/PublicComment/pubcommentPropSub_305.pdf. Accessed January 29, 2014.

21. McGoon MD, Miller DP. REVEAL registry: registry to evaluate early and long-term PAH disease management. 2006. Available at: http://clinicaltrials.gov/show/NCT00370214. Accessed January 29, 2014.

22. Titman A, Rogers CA, Bonser RS, et al. Disease-specific survival benefit of lung transplantation in adults: a National Cohort Study. Am J Transplant 2009;9(7):1640–9.

23. Egan T, Bennett LE, Garrity ER, et al. Predictors of death on the UNOS lung transplant waiting list: results of a multivariate analysis. J Heart Lung Transplant 2001;20(2):242.

24. Charman SC, Sharples LD, McNeil KD, et al. Assessment of survival benefit after lung transplantation by patient diagnosis. J Heart Lung Transplant 2002;21(2):226–32.

25. De Meester J, Smits JM, Persijn GG, et al. Listing for lung transplantation: life expectancy and transplant effect, stratified by type of end-stage lung disease, the Eurotransplant experience. J Heart Lung Transplant 2001;20(5):518–24.

26. McGoon MD, Miller DP. REVEAL: a contemporary US pulmonary arterial hypertension registry. Eur Respir Rev 2012;21(123):8–18.

27. Benza RL, Miller DP, Barst RJ, et al. An evaluation of long-term survival from time of diagnosis in pulmonary arterial hypertension from the REVEAL Registry. Chest 2012;142(2):448–56.

28. Christie JD, Edwards LB, Kucheryavaya AY, et al. The Registry of the International Society for Heart and Lung Transplantation: twenty-seventh official

adult lung and heart-lung transplant report—2010. J Heart Lung Transplant 2010;29(10):1104–18.

29. Schaffer JM, Singh SK, Joyce DL, et al. Transplantation for Idiopathic pulmonary arterial hypertension: improvement in the lung allocation score era. Circulation 2013;127(25):2503–13.

30. Chen H, Shiboski SC, Golden JA, et al. Impact of the lung allocation score on lung transplantation for pulmonary arterial hypertension. Am J Respir Crit Care Med 2009;180(5):468.

31. Galiè N, Ghofrani HA, Torbicki A, et al. Sildenafil citrate therapy for pulmonary arterial hypertension. N Engl J Med 2005;353(20):2148–57.

32. Wilkins MR, Paul GA, Strange JW, et al. Sildenafil versus endothelin receptor antagonist for pulmonary hypertension (SERAPH) study. Am J Respir Crit Care Med 2005;171(11):1292–7.

33. Ghofrani HA, Wiedemann R, Rose F, et al. Combination therapy with oral sildenafil and inhaled iloprost for severe pulmonary hypertension. Ann Intern Med 2002;136(7):515–22.

34. Olschewski H, Simonneau G, Galiè N, et al. Inhaled iloprost for severe pulmonary hypertension. N Engl J Med 2002;347(5):322–9.

35. Kotloff RM, Thabut G. Lung transplantation. Am J Respir Crit Care Med 2011;184(2):159–71.

36. Egan TM. Ethical issues in thoracic organ distribution for transplant. Am J Transplant 2003;3(4):366–72.

37. Thabut G, Christie J, Mal H, et al. Survival benefit of lung transplant for cystic fibrosis since lung-allocation-score implementation. Am J Respir Crit Care Med 2013;187(12):1335–40.

38. O'Beirne S, Counihan IP, Keane MP. Interstitial lung disease and lung transplantation. Semin Respir Crit Care Med 2010;31(2):139–46.

39. Garrity E, Moore J, Mulligan MS, et al. Heart and lung transplantation in the United States, 1996–2005. Am J Transplant 2007;7(S1):1390–403.

40. Whelan TP, Dunity JM, Kelly RF, et al. Effect of preoperative pulmonary artery pressure on early survival after lung transplantation for idiopathic pulmonary fibrosis. J Heart Lung Transplant 2005; 24(9):1269–74.

41. De Oliveira NC, Osaki S, Maloney J, et al. Lung transplant for interstitial lung disease: outcomes before and after implementation of the united network for organ sharing lung allocation scoring system. Eur J Cardiothorac Surg 2012;41(3): 680–5.

42. Orens JB, Shearon TH, Freudenberger RS, et al. Thoracic organ transplantation in the United States, 1995–2004. Am J Transplant 2006;6(5Pt 2):1188–97.

43. Genao L, Whitson HE, Zaas DW, et al. Functional status after lung transplantation in older adults in the post-allocation score era. Am J Transplant 2013;13(1):157–66.

44. Yusen R, Shearon TH, Qian Y, et al. Lung transplantation in the United States, 1999–2008. Am J Transplant 2010;10(4 Pt 2):1047–68.

45. Trulock EP, Edwards LB, Taylor DO, et al. Registry of the International Society for Heart and Lung Transplantation: twenty-second official adult lung and heart-lung transplant report—2005. J Heart Lung Transplant 2005;24(8):956–67.

46. Mahidhara R, Bastani S, Ross DJ, et al. Lung transplantation in older patients? J Thorac Cardiovasc Surg 2008;135(2):412–20.

47. Vadnerkar A, Toyoda Y, Crespo M, et al. Age-specific complications among lung transplant recipients 60 years and older. J Heart Lung Transplant 2011; 30(3):273–81.

48. Kilic A, Merlo CA, Conte JV, et al. Lung transplantation in patients 70 years old or older: have outcomes changed after implementation of the lung allocation score? J Thorac Cardiovasc Surg 2012;144(5):1133–8.

49. Wille KM, Harrington KF, Deandrade JA, et al. Disparities in lung transplantation before and after introduction of the lung allocation score. J Heart Lung Transplant 2013;32(7):684–92.

50. Thabut G, Munson J, Haynes K, et al. Geographic disparities in access to lung transplantation before and after implementation of the lung allocation score. Am J Transplant 2012;12(11):3085–93.

51. Organ Procurement and Transplantation Network. Available at: http://optn.transplant.hrsa.gov. Accessed January 29, 2014.

52. Kozower BD, Meyers BG, Smith MA, et al. The impact of the lung allocation score on short-term transplantation outcomes: a multicenter study. J Thorac Cardiovasc Surg 2008;135(1):166–71.

53. Russo MJ, Iribarne A, Hong KN, et al. High lung allocation score is associated with increased morbidity and mortality following transplantation. Chest 2010; 137(3):651–7.

54. Tsuang WM, Vock DM, Copeland CA, et al. An acute change in lung allocation score and survival after lung transplantation: a cohort study. Ann Intern Med 2013;158(9):650–7.

55. Jackson A, Cropper A, Pye R, et al. Use of extracorporeal membrane oxygenation as a bridge to primary lung transplant: 3 consecutive, successful cases and a review of the literature. J Heart Lung Transplant 2008;27(3):348–52.

56. Nosotti M, Rosso L, Palleschi A, et al. Bridge to lung transplantation by venovenous extracorporeal membrane oxygenation: a lesson learned on the first four cases. Transplant Proc 2010;42(4):1259–61.

57. Olsson K, Simon A, Strueber M, et al. Extracorporeal membrane oxygenation in nonintubated patients as bridge to lung transplantation. Am J Transplant 2010;10(9):2173–8.

58. Turner DA, Cheifetz IM, Rehder KJ; et al. Active rehabilitation and physical therapy during

extracorporeal membrane oxygenation while awaiting lung transplantation: a practical approach. Crit Care Med 2011;39(12):2593–8.

59. Rehder KJ, Turner DA, Hartwig MG, et al. Active rehabilitation during extracorporeal membrane oxygenation as a bridge to lung transplantation. Respir Care 2013;58(8):1291–8.

60. Fuehner T, Kuehn C, Hadem J, et al. Extracorporeal membrane oxygenation in awake patients as bridge to lung transplantation. Am J Respir Crit Care Med 2012;185(7):763–8.

61. Chamogeorgakis T, Mason DP, Murthy SC, et al. Impact of nutritional state on lung transplant outcomes. J Heart Lung Transplant 2013;32(7): 693–700.

62. Allen JG, Arnaoutakis GJ, Weiss ES, et al. The impact of recipient body mass index on survival after lung transplantation. J Heart Lung Transplant 2010;29(9):1026–33.

63. Felker G, Hernandez AF, Rogers JG, et al. Cardiac transplantation at Duke UniversityMedical Center. Clin Transpl 2003;18:235–41.

64. McCue JD, Mooney J, Quail J, et al. Ninety-day mortality and major complications are not affected by use of lung allocation score. J Heart Lung Transplant 2008;27(2):192–6.

65. Hachem RR, Trulock EP. The new lung allocation system and its impact on waitlist characteristics and post-transplant outcomes. Semin Thorac Cardiovasc Surg 2008;20(2):139–42. Elsevier. WB Saunders.

ECMO as Bridge to Lung Transplant

Mauer Biscotti, MD, Joshua Sonett, MD*, Matthew Bacchetta, MD

KEYWORDS

• ECMO • Lung transplant • Bridge to transplant

KEY POINTS

- Extracorporeal membrane oxygenation (ECMO) can be safely used for extended periods of time to optimize critically ill patients.
- ECMO as a bridge to transplantation (BTT) can be effective when extensive preoperative planning and stringent daily clinical assessment are used.
- ECMO can be used as a means to optimize patients with physical therapy.
- Posttransplant outcomes of patients on ECMO for BTT are acceptable.
- Larger studies and refined decision algorithms are necessary to optimize patient outcomes.

INTRODUCTION
History of Lung Transplantation

The first lung transplant was performed in 1963 by Dr James Hardy, and after decades of refining both the surgical technique and postoperative medical management, it is now the standard of care for select, end-stage diseases of the lung.[1] Although there have been great advances in lung transplantation, it still comprises only 4% of the organs transplanted in the United States. Additionally, mortality outcomes for lung transplantation are not as good as for other solid organs, likely due to higher rates of infection, rejection, impaired anastomotic healing, and chronic rejection in the form of bronchiolitis obliterans.

Lung Allocation Score

Until 2005, the allocation of lungs was based on waiting list time. This meant that patients before 2005 would receive lungs purely based on length of time on the waiting list and not on medical necessity or predicted posttransplant outcomes. However, beginning in 2005, both medical urgency

and net benefit from transplantation were incorporated to create a standardized scoring system from 0 to 100.[1] This change in the lung-allocation process has decreased the total number of patients on the waiting list, decreased total waiting time, and reduced the death rate in patients on the waiting list.[1]

Factors affecting Lung Allocation Score
There are multiple factors incorporated into the Lung Allocation Score (LAS), with underlying disease being given the most weight. These factors were demarcated into 2 groups: Waiting List Survival and Predicted Posttransplant Survival. Age, forced vital capacity, oxygen requirements, functional status, 6-minute walk distance, diagnosis, and mechanical ventilation are some of the factors currently used in calculating LAS.[2]

Pretransplant mechanical ventilation
Since the adoption of the current LAS system, patients receiving continuous mechanical ventilation receive higher scores, meaning they are more likely to receive a transplant. However, issues related to ventilator-dependent patient

Disclosure: None.
Section of Thoracic Surgery, Price Family Center for Comprehensive Chest Care, Center for Acute Respiratory Care, Columbia University Medical Center, New York–Presbyterian Hospital, 161 Fort Washington Avenue, 3rd Floor, New York, NY 10032, USA
* Corresponding author.
E-mail address: js2106@columbia.edu

conditioning, and posttransplantation survival, have given pause to transplantation centers. It has been hypothesized that patients receiving continuous mechanical ventilation before transplantation may be too sick for transplantation, which may affect posttransplant outcomes. This issue was studied in 2010, and posttransplant survival in patients receiving pretransplant mechanical ventilation was found to be significantly lower than unsupported patients.[3] Although survival was worse in these patients at 1 year (57% vs 70% for unsupported patients), it was not considered prohibitive. Additionally, after 6 months, the survival curves of patients receiving mechanical ventilation before transplantation versus unsupported patients were comparable, suggesting most of the increase in mortality risk was in the immediate postoperative period.

Pretransplant physical therapy/conditioning

Patients with a lung transplant, even with relatively normal postoperative pulmonary function tests and gas exchange, have decreased postoperative exercise capacity. These patients appear to have limited peripheral muscle aerobic capacity and peak muscle force.[4] Additionally, there is a weak correlation between postoperative exercise capacity and length of time spent on the waiting list, which suggests that preoperative deconditioning plays a role.[4] Nearly all patients will show a decline in skeletal muscle function postoperatively, regardless of the extent of pretransplant dysfunction.[5] Although the evidence points toward a postoperative decline in skeletal muscle function, this loss could be mitigated by improving the preoperative physical condition of the patient with better preservation of skeletal muscle function. Although a direct causal relationship between participation in a preoperative rehabilitation program and postoperative exercise tolerance has not been established, it is generally considered a standard of care to enlist all patients into a pulmonary rehabilitation program before transplantation. Given the belief that pretransplant conditioning will prove beneficial to posttransplant outcomes, patients who are bridged to transplant on extracorporeal membrane oxygenation (ECMO) now undergo active pulmonary rehabilitation at some centers.[6] There appears to be a benefit from pretransplant pulmonary rehabilitation even in this select group of extremely sick patients, despite the paucity of data.[6]

History of Extracorporeal Membrane Oxygenation

ECMO has been used for the treatment of refractory respiratory or cardiac failure for more than 4 decades now. Through continuously improving technology and extensive clinical experience, ECMO has evolved from a novelty at a select few centers to a routine practice at more than 200 centers internationally. With the Conventional Ventilatory Support Versus Extracorporeal Membrane Oxygenation for Severe Adult Respiratory Failure (CESAR) trial and the outbreak of influenza A H1N1-associated severe acute respiratory distress syndrome (ARDS) in 2009, ECMO has become a rapidly growing modality of support in many tertiary care medical centers.[7,8] ECMO is now used to support patients suffering from neonatal cardiac and respiratory failure, postcardiotomy shock, post cardiac arrest, and ARDS; as a bridge to heart and/or lung transplantation; and in the transport of critically ill patients among others.[9]

Types of extracorporeal membrane oxygenation

Typical ECMO configurations are venovenous (VV) and venoarterial (VA), which provide respiratory and combined respiratory and circulatory support, respectively. In VV ECMO, blood is withdrawn and returned to the central venous system after passing through a pump and oxygenator system, thereby delivering oxygenated blood to the right atrium. This can be done with either a dual-site or single-site configuration. In VA ECMO, blood is withdrawn from a central vein and returned to a large-caliber peripheral or central artery, providing both hemodynamic and respiratory support.

In patients receiving VV ECMO who develop refractory cardiac dysfunction, an arterial limb can be spliced into the reinfusion circuit, creating a VVA ECMO system, which augments both pulmonary and cardiac function. Additionally, in patients receiving VA ECMO who develop severely compromised native gas exchange, an additional oxygenated venous reinfusion cannula can be branched from the arterial tubing and inserted into a jugular vein, thereby delivering oxygenated blood to the right heart and, in turn, to the coronary and carotid circulations, creating a VA-V ECMO circuit. These configurations can be useful before lung transplantation in patients who have intrinsic lung disease and develop secondary right heart dysfunction.

What Is a Bridge?

With the scarcity of organs suitable for transplantation and an increase in the number of patients on transplant waiting lists, the need for a device to "bridge" patients who were otherwise failing optimal medical management became more apparent. Beginning in 1969 with the first bridge to cardiac transplantation by Cooley, followed by the technological refinements and increased clinical experience with left ventricular assist devices (LVADs), a "bridge to transplant" (BTT) became a reality for primary cardiac disease. Although LVADs were predominantly used for postcardiotomy cardiogenic shock in their infancy, they have recently been used to bridge failing patients to heart transplantation with excellent success compared with non–mechanically assisted patients.[10,11] Taking direction from the success in bridging of patients with heart failure using mechanical support, several lung transplant programs have used ECMO to bridge failing transplant candidates in recent years.

Past bridge-to-transplant experience

Beginning in 2005, the University of Pittsburgh Medical Center began using ECMO as a BTT for patients before lung transplantation. Over a 6-year period, they used ECMO as a bridge in 31 patients, with 25 ultimately surviving to transplantation. Of the patients successfully bridged, they demonstrated a 74% 2-year survival compared with 74% for unsupported patients. The rate of primary graft dysfunction (PGD) requiring posttransplant ECMO was higher in the BTT group, but based on graft survival, they demonstrated efficacy using ECMO as BTT.[12]

The University of Kentucky and University of California San Francisco also have used ECMO as a BTT for lung transplantation and they have successfully bridged 31 patients as of 2013. They have achieved similar success, demonstrating 80% 3-year survival in patients bridged with ECMO, which compares favorably with a registry of similarly ill transplant patients. Of the 31 patients who they successfully bridged, 19 were ambulatory at the time of transplantation, which demonstrates one of the benefits of bridging extremely debilitated patients using ECMO.[13]

A group from France reported their experience in which 36 people were placed on ECMO as a bridge, with 30 patients ultimately receiving a lung transplant. Of these 30 patients, the 2-year survival rate was 60.5% overall. The survival in this study was lower than in the previously described series. However, they demonstrated a significant survival advantage for patients with cystic fibrosis (CF) compared with idiopathic pulmonary fibrosis (IPF) among patients bridged (71% vs 27.3%, respectively).[14] These data suggest there may be differences in outcome and "supportability" based on etiology of lung disease.

A retrospective analysis from 2 centers in Italy hinted that length of duration on ECMO as a BTT

has an effect on survival and morbidity after transplantation. They demonstrated a 76% 1-year survival after transplantation in patients who received BTT; however, they noted that an ECMO bridge less than 14 days compared with longer than 14 days conferred a sizable survival advantage.[15] However, the study did not clearly elucidate the physiologic status of the patients before transplantation nor did it outline the means of determining or maintaining transplant eligibility while on ECMO.

Extracorporeal Membrane Oxygenation as a Bridge to Transplantation

We published our experience with ECMO as BTT in 2012. At that time, we had a 5-year experience with using ECMO as a bridge for 18 patients. Of those 18 patients, 10 received lung transplantation, 3 returned to baseline function and were decannulated, and 5 died during the bridge. Of the 10 patients who received lung transplantation all were alive at 3 months and of the 6 patients who were 1-year posttransplant, all were alive as well.

Decision-making before extracorporeal membrane oxygenation

Since our first successful BTT in 2007, we have gained experience and refined our pre-ECMO decision-making process. Our multidisciplinary team consists of lung transplant pulmonologists, ECMO intensivists, a surgical ECMO specialist-transplant surgeon, and critical care intensivists. Our multidisciplinary ECMO-transplant team discusses all patients at our institution who are listed for lung transplantation and admitted to the hospital for worsening respiratory status. Among the most important factors used to decide whether a patient will benefit from a BTT are age, functional status, underlying disease, infection, other organ dysfunction, and anticipated time on the waitlist.

In our experience, younger patients and those patients who have been actively participating in a pulmonary rehabilitation program with a good functional status before admission are those who fare best on ECMO as a BTT. Because the BTT ECMO run can last beyond a week in many patients, we attempt to select patients who will be active participants in physical therapy while in the intensive care unit. Given that, the timing of placing a patient on ECMO is paramount. It is important to select patients who have not decompensated to the point that post-ECMO rehabilitation will be impossible. Patients must demonstrate a true progression of disease that shows no realistic chance of improvement, but who also have enough physical reserve left to be an active participant in their own pretransplant rehabilitation. Participation in physical therapy remains a critical metric that the ECMO and transplant teams use to assess the ongoing transplant eligibility of BTT patients.

Infection is another important factor when considering appropriate BTT candidates. Active, culture-proven bloodstream infections are a relative contraindication to placing patients on ECMO, as the long-term indwelling venous or arterial cannulas will be at risk for seeding with bacteria and remain a source of infection. Additionally, pulmonary infections with certain bacteria, such as highly resistant *Achromobacter* species, are a relative contraindication. These gram-negative bacteria produce a biofilm, which makes post-transplant infections very difficult to treat. Finally, patients with other moderate to severe organ dysfunction, including renal, liver, and left ventricular failure that is unrelated to their primary lung dysfunction (ie, hypoxemia, hypercapnia, or secondary pulmonary hypertension) are not considered candidates for BTT because of their baseline increased risk.

Family and patient discussions are one of the most important aspects of the pre-ECMO BTT decision-making process. Expectations must be clearly set, such that if the patient develops other end-organ failure, becomes incapable of participating in physical therapy, cannot meet nutritional requirements, or continues to deteriorate physiologically and suffers severe debilitation even after initiation of ECMO, then transplant eligibility will be called into question. It is the responsibility of the transplant team to continually assess the patient's transplant status to ensure optimal survival and use of scarce donor organs. If the patient is no longer deemed a transplant candidate, then the use of ECMO as a BTT will be withheld in a manner suitable to the patient and family.

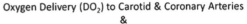

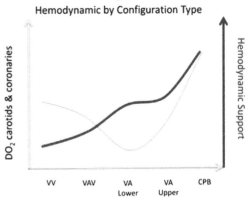

Fig. 1. Level of support by configuration type. CPB, cardiopulmonary bypass; DO$_2$, oxygen delivery. (*From* Biscotti M, Lee A, Basner RC, et al. Hybrid configurations via percutaneous access for extracorporeal membrane oxygenation: a single center experience. ASAIO J 2014;60; with permission.)

Surgical considerations

After a patient is deemed a suitable candidate for ECMO-BTT, the ideal surgical approach must be considered. The ECMO circuit can be configured in multiple ways, such as VV, VA, or VVA, with peripheral or central access depending on the underlying disease and pathophysiology of that particular patient (**Fig. 1, Table 1**). The type of configuration chosen should correct the patient's underlying pathophysiologic state, afford optimal mobility, and provide simplicity for bedside management.

Patients without significant right heart dysfunction, with hypercapnic, hypoxemic, or combined respiratory failure, typically benefit best from VV ECMO. Most patients with CF are young, with preserved right and left ventricular function, and simply need VV ECMO to sweep off CO_2 and to

Table 1
Hybrid extracorporeal membrane oxygenation configuration characteristics

	VV	VV with ASD	VA Femoral	VA Upper Body	VAV	PA-LA
DO$_2$	+++	+++	Lower: ++++ Upper: +	++++	+++	++++
mPAP	(−)	Marginal	++++	++++	++	+++
RV support	+	++	++++	++++	+++	+++
Patient mobility	++++	++++	(−)	++++	Lower: (−) Upper: ++++	+++
Simplicity	++++	+++	+++	++	+++	+

Abbreviations: +, minimal; ++, moderate; +++, good; ++++, excellent; (−), no advantage; ASD, atrial septal defect; DO$_2$, delivery of oxygen; mPAP, mean pulmonary artery pressure; PA-LA, pulmonary artery to left atrium; RV, right ventricle; VA, venoarterial; VAV, venoarterial-venous; VV, venovenous.

improve oxygenation. In our experience, single-site VV ECMO using the Avalon Elite Bicaval Dual Lumen cannula (Maquet, Rastatt, Germany) is well suited for these patients (**Fig. 2**). Although VV ECMO can be dual-site or single-site, the single-site configuration with insertion into the right or left internal jugular vein provides freedom from groin cannulation and allows patients to ambulate without the risks associated with femoral cannulation.

In patients with progressive respiratory failure, but who have significant right heart strain from either primary or secondary pulmonary hypertension, VV ECMO is often insufficient to provide adequate support. In these patients, typically with IPF or idiopathic pulmonary artery hypertension (IPAH), VA ECMO or a pulmonary artery–to–left atrium circuit is the configuration of choice. We prefer to avoid central cannulation when possible to simplify the approach at the time of transplantation. Although VA ECMO is historically instituted via femoral arteries and veins, this is suboptimal in patients who we expect to participate in physical therapy. Furthermore, the retrograde flow from the femoral artery will not deliver good oxygenation to the upper body, specifically the carotid and coronary arteries. As such, we prefer to use an upper-body VA ECMO configuration in these patients. The right internal jugular vein is used for drainage with a 23-Fr arterial Biomedicus cannula (Medtronic, Brooklyn Park, MN), while the right subclavian artery is surgically cannulated.[16] Depending on the size of the subclavian artery, either a 6-mm or 8-mm Hemashield graft is sewn at a sharply beveled angle and tunneled laterally with either an 18-Fr or 24-Fr Elongated One-Piece Arterial (EOPA) cannula (Medtronic) inserted in a sleevelike fashion (**Fig. 3**). This configuration provides adequate oxygenation to the upper body and lower body

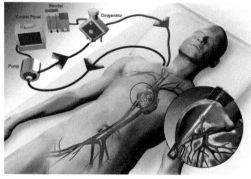

Fig. 2. Single-site dual-lumen VV ECMO configuration. (*Reprinted with permission* from CollectedMed.com, Columbia University Medical Center, New York, NY.)

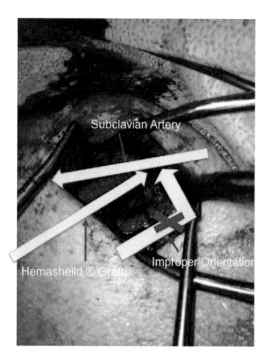

Fig. 3. "Sport-Model" graft-subclavian artery anastomosis.

in addition to decompressing the strained right ventricle.

A subset of patients on VV ECMO for BTT will continue to develop progressive right heart failure during the bridge. These patients can benefit from a reconfiguration, by splicing an arterial reinfusion limb into the circuit. This setup is then termed VVA ECMO. This occurs most commonly in the older patients with IPF. The arterial reinfusion limb is placed as described previously, in an upper body configuration. Drainage remains through the internal jugular vein, and oxygenated blood reinfusion is via both the internal jugular vein and the right subclavian artery. This configuration decompresses the right heart and provides oxygenated blood through both the native pulmonary circulation and into the subclavian artery (**Fig. 4**). It will often require placement of a partial clamping device on the internal jugular limb to balance the oxygenated return flow between the low-pressure central venous system and the systemic arterial circulation (**Fig. 5**).

An important surgical consideration when placing patients on ECMO for BTT is the necessity or timing of tracheostomy. We prefer early tracheostomy for patients whom we believe need aggressive pulmonary toilet, who have already been intubated for more than 1 week, or who subsequently develop the need for ventilatory support

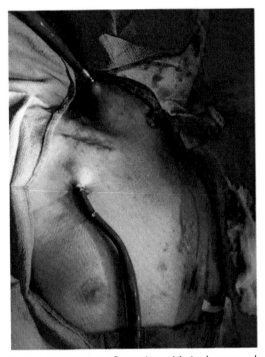

Fig. 4. VVA ECMO configuration with Avalon cannula and subclavian artery reinfusion limb.

to ease their work of breathing. Patients who are intubated at the time of decision to place them on ECMO typically benefit from early tracheostomy, especially if it can be performed safely,

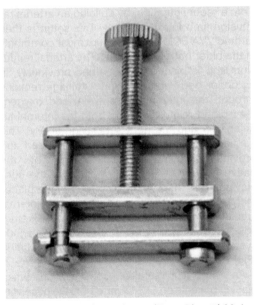

Fig. 5. Hoffman tubing clamp. (*From* Biscotti M, Lee A, Basner RC, et al. Hybrid configurations via percutaneous access for extracorporeal membrane oxygenation: a single center experience. ASAIO J 2014;60; with permission.)

before initiating ECMO and giving heparin boluses. When a tracheostomy and ECMO cannulation are done at the same time, we prefer to perform the ECMO cannulation first, so as not to lose the airway and risk a hypoxemic or hypercapnic arrest. Because we often do the tracheostomy after cannulation and a heparin bolus, we give a bolus of aminocaproic acid followed by a 6-hour infusion at half normal dosage. Although we usually perform percutaneous tracheostomies, we use electrocautery to dissect through the skin and superficial subcutaneous tissue to mitigate any future bleeding complications. As we do with our ECMO cannulation sites, a pursestring of 3-0 nylon suture is placed around the tracheostomy to tamponade oozing from the incision.

After deciding on the ECMO configuration, the next step is to choose the appropriate cannula size and type. For standard VV ECMO, we prefer the Avalon cannula (Maquet), which facilitates easier patient mobilization. If patients have purely hypercapnic failure, the amount of blood flow required to adequately support them is much less than if they have hypoxemic failure as well. For this reason, we first calculate the patient's anticipated cardiac output for a cardiac index of 2.4 L/min/m^2 and estimate his or her oxygen demands. When a patient has hypoxemic failure, or we anticipate a progression to severe hypoxemic failure, we attempt to place a cannula that is of sufficient size to match his or her entire cardiac output. The Avalon cannula flows in vivo are typically 2.5 L/min for a 23-Fr, 4 L/min for a 27-Fr, and up to 5 L/min for a 31-Fr cannula. When a patient has purely hypercapnic failure and their oxygenation is not problematic, we will use a 23-Fr or 27-Fr Avalon cannula.

For the upper-body "Sport Model" VA ECMO configuration, the cannula size is more standardized. We use a 23-Fr Arterial Biomedicus (Medtronic) for drainage. We do not use a venous cannula for drainage because the cannula is much longer than the arterial cannula, which makes neck cannulation more cumbersome. The reinfusion cannula is either an 18-Fr or 24-Fr EOPA (Medtronic) based on the size of the patient's subclavian artery and the use of either a 6-mm or 8-mm graft.

In our experience, many of these patients who receive ECMO as a BTT will require support for 1 week or longer, and infection risk reduction is paramount. For this reason, we dress our ECMO cannulation sites with a chlorhexidine-impregnated dressing. The dressing is changed under sterile conditions and cleaned with a chlorhexidine swab every third day. Additionally, we use a very simple ECMO circuit, consisting of drainage cannula, centrifugal pump, oxygenator, and reinfusion cannula. We have preoxygenator and postoxygenator pressure tubing attached to monitor the transoxygenator pressure gradient, but no other connections are spliced into the circuit to reduce inadvertent contamination. With meticulous cannula site care and minimal circuit connections, our bloodstream infection rate has remained extremely low.

Extracorporeal membrane oxygenation course

The ultimate goal of using ECMO as a BTT is to halt the progression of debilitation and make candidates more robust before transplantation to ensure the best possible posttransplant outcomes. A key step is to engage these patients with physical therapy as early and as often as possible. With optimal cannulation configurations and improved physiology, patients receiving BTT should have the capacity to work with physical therapy daily, meet their caloric needs, and gain strength. Beginning as early as ECMO day 1, we mobilize our patients receiving BTT out of bed to chair, if possible, and often begin walking less than 24 hours after cannulation. Our physical therapy team, in conjunction with perfusionists, nurse practitioners, ECMO specialists, and nurses all participate in a highly coordinated effort to move the patient, ECMO system, and ventilator, if needed.[17] Physical therapy is continued daily until the time of transplantation. Several patients have been able to walk more than 1500 feet with minimal assistance and rest during their bridge (**Fig. 6**).

One difference in the management of patients receiving BTT ECMO compared with patients receiving standard ECMO is ventilator weaning. We only wean the ventilator, Fio_2, high-flow nasal cannula, or other forms of supplemental oxygen if the patient continues to remain comfortable.

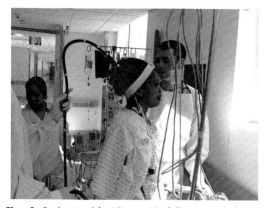

Fig. 6. Patient with "Sport Model" as BTT during ambulation. (*Courtesy of* New York Presbyterian/Columbia University Medical Center, New York, NY.)

Unlike in ARDS or other indications for oxygen therapy, there is no imperative to wean Fio_2, because the patient is on a pathway of transplantation and not recovery of native lung function. We target optimal ECMO blood flow and sweep gas flow in addition to supplemental oxygen to enable the patients to participate fully in their pretransplant rehabilitation. To this end, it is not uncommon for us to maintain our patients receiving ECMO on 100% Fio_2 as needed to keep them comfortable during physical therapy.

With our patients receiving standard ECMO, we use a very conservative transfusion policy. We will transfuse packed red blood cells only if the hemoglobin is lower than 7 g/dL or if the patient remains persistently hypoxemic (SpO_2 <92%) despite maximal ECMO settings. In the patients receiving BTT, the transfusion policy is even more conservative. Unless there are hemodynamic or end-organ perfusion issues from anemia, the patient cannot work with physical therapy, or if the hemoglobin is persistently lower than 6 g/dL, we will prohibit transfusion to reduce the risk of eliciting an antibody response that may adversely affect their organ cross-match profile.

Clinicians are presented with a difficult medical and ethical decision when patients fail to thrive on ECMO BTT; that is, when patients are unable to participate in their own rehabilitation and have continued to fail physiologically despite maximal extracorporeal support. In our program, the patient receiving ECMO BTT is reviewed every day for maintenance of transplant suitability. If the patient develops renal failure, liver failure, left ventricular failure, sepsis, or does not get out of bed for more than 7 days, he or she will be de-listed because it is highly unlikely the patient will do well posttransplantation. If the decision is made to de-list the patient from the lung transplant waiting list, a family meeting is held to discuss withdrawal of support. Once there is no option for lung transplantation in these end-stage patients, ECMO becomes a bridge to nowhere. The lung and ECMO teams hold meetings with the patient and family to determine the timing and manner of withdrawal of support (**Fig. 7**).

Transplant on extracorporeal membrane oxygenation

All patients who are bridged to transplant on ECMO will remain on ECMO throughout the eventual lung transplant operation unless they need a cardiac procedure, such as atrial septal defect (ASD) closure, at which point they are switched to cardiopulmonary bypass. At the completion of the procedure, an attempt at weaning ECMO is performed in the operating room unless patients

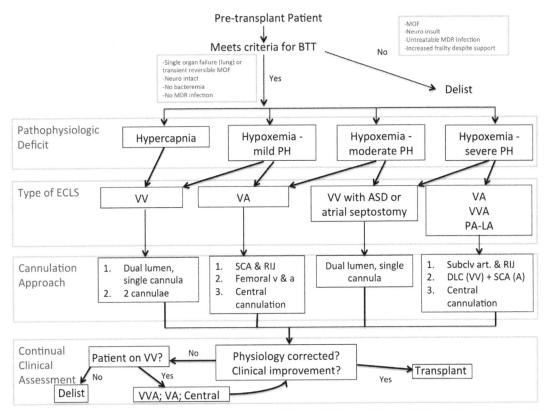

Fig. 7. Decision algorithm. DLC, double lumen cannula; MDR, multidrug resistant; MOF, multiorgan failure; PA-LA, pulmonary artery to left atrium; PH, pulmonary hypertension; RIJ, right internal jugular vein; SCA, subclavian artery.

continue to demonstrate hemodynamic instability or hypoxemic/hypercapneic respiratory failure. In our experience, 31.6% of patients bridged to transplant with ECMO may require continuation of ECMO postoperatively.

Outcomes

Given the severity of their underlying disease process and frequent LAS greater than 90, patients receiving ECMO BTT have a higher than expected mortality. We have placed 43 patients on ECMO for BTT. Twenty-one of these patients had CF, 12 had IPF, 6 had IPAH, 2 had chronic obstructive pulmonary disease, 1 had emphysema, and 1 had bronchiectasis. Of these, 32 had VV ECMO, 8 had VA ECMO, 2 had VVA ECMO, and 1 had central cannulation. Of the 43 patients, 25 patients ambulated with physical therapy before transplantation. A total of 23 patients (53.5%) were successfully bridged to transplant, which is a modest rate; however, 20 of these patients (87.0%) survived to discharge. One-year survival for those at risk was 85.7%, with a mean follow-up of 21 months, which is consistent with the outcomes of Hoopes and colleagues.[13]

Contrary to some previous studies, there was no statistically significant difference between duration of ECMO support for patients who died versus those who were successfully transplanted. Our experience confirms that ECMO can be used to successfully bridge critically ill patients to lung transplantation. Additionally, of the patients who continued to meet transplant criteria and were successfully transplanted, postoperative survival rates are comparable with patients not receiving mechanical circulatory support.

Future Directions

Creating a multicenter database to identify relevant clinical factors to optimize the methods of support and clinical parameters to assess the patient's ongoing transplant suitability will inform the decision-making algorithms for lung BTT. Excellent outcomes can be achieved, but it is imperative that larger studies be performed to inform decision algorithms for BTT and to optimize outcomes. Cost analysis of ECMO per life gained has not been performed and can be challenging in this diverse cohort of patients; however, we must be mindful of the significant costs incurred by

EMCO. However, using ECMO in a team-driven decision analysis, instituting and terminating BTT selectively and prospectively, will help keep this resource-heavy intervention cost-effective in terms of life years gained. Earlier introduction of ECMO, before irreversible debilitation and persistent frailty, will likely improve the success and costs of bridging patients.

Despite the challenges of ECMO BTT, this experience will likely provide the prerequisite step in the development of more long-term and durable support systems for patients requiring lung transplantation in the same vein as the early LVAD experience did for bridging to heart transplantation and destination therapy. A long-term paracorporeal lung-assist device and ultimately an artificial lung could potentially provide support for months to years in patients with end-stage lung disease.

REFERENCES

1. Kotloff RM, Thabut G. Lung transplantation. Am J Respir Crit Care Med 2011;184:159–71.
2. Egan TM, Murray S, Bustami RT, et al. Development of the new lung allocation system in the United States. Am J Transplant 2006;6:1212–27.
3. Mason DP, Thuita L, Nowicki ER, et al. Should lung transplantation be performed for patients on mechanical respiratory support? The US experience. J Thorac Cardiovasc Surg 2010;139:765–73.e1.
4. Maury G, Langer D, Verleden G, et al. Skeletal muscle force and functional exercise tolerance before and after lung transplantation: a cohort study. Am J Transplant 2008;8:1275–81.
5. Reinsma GD, ten Hacken NH, Grevink RG, et al. Limiting factors of exercise performance 1 year after lung transplantation. J Heart Lung Transplant 2006;25:1310–6.
6. Rehder KJ, Turner DA, Hartwig MG, et al. Active rehabilitation during extracorporeal membrane oxygenation as a bridge to lung transplantation. Respir Care 2013;58:1291–8.
7. Brodie D, Bacchetta M. Extracorporeal membrane oxygenation for ARDS in adults. N Engl J Med 2011;365:1905–14.
8. Peek GJ, Mugford M, Tiruvoipati R, et al. Efficacy and economic assessment of conventional ventilatory support versus extracorporeal membrane oxygenation for severe adult respiratory failure (CESAR): a multicentre randomised controlled trial. Lancet 2009;374:1351–63.
9. Bartlett RH, Roloff DW, Custer JR, et al. Extracorporeal life support: the University of Michigan experience. JAMA 2000;283:904–8.
10. Arabia FA, Smith RG, Rose DS, et al. Success rates of long-term circulatory assist devices used currently for bridge to heart transplantation. ASAIO J 1996;42:M542–6.
11. Birks EJ, Yacoub MH, Banner NR, et al. The role of bridge to transplantation: should LVAD patients be transplanted? Curr Opin Cardiol 2004;19:148–53.
12. Toyoda Y, Bhama JK, Shigemura N, et al. Efficacy of extracorporeal membrane oxygenation as a bridge to lung transplantation. J Thorac Cardiovasc Surg 2013;145:1065–70 [discussion: 1070–1].
13. Hoopes CW, Kukreja J, Golden J, et al. Extracorporeal membrane oxygenation as a bridge to pulmonary transplantation. J Thorac Cardiovasc Surg 2013;145:862–7 [discussion: 867–8].
14. Lafarge M, Mordant P, Thabut G, et al. Experience of extracorporeal membrane oxygenation as a bridge to lung transplantation in France. J Heart Lung Transplant 2013;32:905–13.
15. Crotti S, Iotti GA, Lissoni A, et al. Organ allocation waiting time during extracorporeal bridge to lung transplant affects outcomes. Chest 2013;144:1018–25.
16. Javidfar J, Brodie D, Costa J, et al. Subclavian artery cannulation for venoarterial extracorporeal membrane oxygenation. ASAIO J 2012;58:494–8.
17. Abrams D, Javidfar J, Farrand E, et al. Early mobilization of patients receiving extracorporeal membrane oxygenation: a retrospective cohort study. Critical Care 2014;18:R38.

Extending the Donor Pool
Rehabilitation of Poor Organs

Marcelo Cypel, MD, MSc[a], Shaf Keshavjee, MD, MSc, FRCSC, FACS[b],*

KEYWORDS

- Lung transplantation • Organ preservation • Ex vivo lung perfusion

KEY POINTS

- Donor lung shortage is a significant limitation in lung transplantation. Only about 20% of lungs from multiorgan donors are used because of injuries occurring during the mechanism of death and intensive care unit–related complications.
- Normothermic ex vivo lung perfusion (EVLP) can significantly improve utilization of donor lungs by improving organ evaluation and by allowing treatment interventions during the ex vivo phase of organ preservation.
- Many clinical trials are underway using different EVLP systems and techniques and the role of normothermic preservation for both standard and extended criteria donor lungs are being investigated.

INTRODUCTION

Lung transplantation (LTx) is a lifesaving therapy for patients with end-stage lung diseases. However, the number of patients waiting for LTx greatly exceeds the number of donors available. A further aggravating factor specific to LTx is that only 15% to 20% of lungs from multiorgan brain death donors (BDDs) are currently deemed usable for clinical transplantation.[1] That number is even smaller (in the range of 2% in the United States) from donors after cardiac death (DCD).[2] Most potential lungs are considered unsuitable because of the lung injury that occurs with brain death and intensive care unit (ICU)–related complications (ie, barotrauma or lung edema associated with fluid resuscitation).[3] Because primary graft dysfunction (PGD) is a complication that leads to severe early and long-term consequences to LTx recipients, transplant teams tend to be conservative in selection of donor lungs. As a result, wait list mortality

generally is as high as 30%.[4,5] A novel strategy to overcome the shortage of lungs is ex vivo lung perfusion (EVLP). EVLP can increase the number of donor lungs available in 2 important ways: (1) better evaluation of questionable organs, and (2) treatment and repair of injured organs. This article focuses on the rationale, recent developments, and current and future potential of normothermic EVLP.

DONOR LUNG PRESERVATION

The current clinical practice of organ preservation is cold static preservation. During retrieval, a cold pulmonary flush using a low-potassium dextran preservation solution is coupled with topical cooling and lung ventilation.[6,7] Lungs are then transported at 4°C in a static inflated state. Hypothermia reduces metabolic activity to the point that cell viability can be maintained despite ischemia (5% of metabolic rate at 37°C).[8] Aerobic cold

Disclosures: M. Cypel and S. Keshavjee are founders of Perfusix. They also received research support from XVIVO Perfusion Inc.
[a] Division of Thoracic Surgery, University of Toronto, 200 Elizabeth Street, 9N-969, Toronto, Ontario M5G 2C4, Canada; [b] Toronto Lung Transplant Program, Division of Thoracic Surgery, University of Toronto, 200 Elizabeth Street, 9N-946, Toronto, Ontario M5G 2C4, Canada
* Corresponding author.
E-mail address: shaf.keshavjee@uhn.ca

Thorac Surg Clin 25 (2015) 27–33
http://dx.doi.org/10.1016/j.thorsurg.2014.09.002
1547-4127/15/$ – see front matter © 2015 Elsevier Inc. All rights reserved.

temperature preservation is therefore still the foundation of lung preservation.[9,10] However, although protective, the main limitation of hypothermic preservation is the significant decrease in organ metabolic functions, which precludes the possibility of meaningful lung evaluation and recovery after the time of organ retrieval.[8]

DEVELOPMENT OF EX VIVO LUNG PERFUSION

It would be ideal for further evaluation and treatment of donor lungs to be possible during the ex vivo phase of the organ, before transplantation into the recipient. In order to achieve this, organ preservation needs to occur at normothermic or near-normothermic conditions so that metabolic functions are preserved. One such strategy has been EVLP. This strategy attempts to simulate the in vivo situation by ventilation and perfusion of the donor lung graft. Originally proposed as early as 1935 by Carrel and Lindbergh[11] for organs in general and then in 1970 by Jirsch and colleagues[12] for the evaluation and preservation of lungs in cases of distant procurement, attempts in those eras failed because of an inability to maintain the air/fluid barrier within the lung, leading to the development of edema and increased pulmonary vascular resistance (PVR) in the donor lung during EVLP.

MODERN ERA OF EX VIVO LUNG PERFUSION

Driven by the objective of achieving an evaluation of the lungs from uncontrolled DCDs in which in vivo evaluation is not possible, Steen and colleagues[13] developed an ex vivo perfusion system with the intent of short-term evaluation. In doing so, they developed a buffered, extracellular solution with an optimized colloid osmotic pressure to act as the lung perfusate (Steen Solution, XVIVO Perfusion, Sweden). This solution helps hold fluid within the intravascular space during perfusion and provides nutrients needed to maintain lung viability for several hours. They used this solution mixed with red blood cells in combination with their circuit and were able to successfully perfuse and evaluate lungs in a large animal model for 1 hour without the development of pulmonary edema, and subsequently achieved successful transplantation.[14] Following work in large animals, Steen and colleagues[15] published a case report of successful transplantation of a nonacceptable lung following a brief period of EVLP in 2007.

The ultimate goal of Steen's studies was to use EVLP as a method for lung evaluation and thus the perfusion times were short (60 minutes). Many similar studies followed in Europe in the same DCD evaluation context.[16–18] For the application of EVLP for preservation, improved evaluation, and the advanced goals of lung recovery and repair, more time is required. Erasmus and colleagues[19] first attempted to extend the EVLP duration to 6 hours; however, circuit-induced injury again became evident with increased PVR and airway pressures in the lung near the end of 6 hours.

In 2008, our group in Toronto was the first to describe the feasibility of stable long-term (12 hours) normothermic EVLP using a lung protective strategy for acellular normothermic perfusion and ventilation; a strategy well known today as the Toronto EVLP method.[20] To obtain stable extended (>12 hours perfusion), several key lung protective strategies were used, such as the use of an acellular solution (Steen solution), protective perfusion flows (40% cardiac output), and a positive physiologic left atrium pressure. Maintenance of a positive left atrial (LA) pressure of 3 to 5 mm Hg was important for the success of long-term perfusion. This small but positive LA pressure tents open the capillaries and postcapillary venules and prevents collapse of the microvessels during increases in airway pressures and decreases of flow at inspiration.[21] Absence of positive LA pressures can lead to unstable alveolar geometry and results in decreased lung compliance.[22] Using this strategy, reproducible, safe 12-hour normothermic ex vivo perfusion has been achieved in porcine and human lungs and it has been shown to interrupt ischemic damage caused by prolonged cold ischemia.[20,23,24]

After these publications, an expansion of EVLP research has occurred, and EVLP became one of the major topics of research in LTx. As expected, in parallel with this success, there has been heightened interest from industry in related technology, with various different companies producing devices for lung perfusion, each with notably different characteristics (discussed later). Several prospective studies of various EVLP techniques are underway or have recently been completed in Europe and North America, including the HELP (Human Ex Vivo Lung Perfusion) trial (Toronto; sponsor XVIVO Perfusion), the NOVEL trial (United States; sponsor XVIVO Perfusion), the INSPIRE and EXPAND trial (Europe and United States; sponsor Transmedics), the DEVELOP UK (United Kingdom; sponsor Vivoline), the Vienna trial (Vienna, sponsor XVIVO), and the Perfusix Trial (United States; sponsor Perfusix). Important differences between these studies (besides the different technologies and techniques) are the specific indications. Although the HELP, NOVEL, Develop UK,

EXPAND, and Perfusix trials include extended criteria lungs, the INSPIRE and Vienna trial are evaluating the impact of EVLP in standard criteria donor lungs. **Table 1** shows completed and ongoing clinical trials using EVLP technology.

EX VIVO LUNG EVALUATION

Current donor lung evaluation is a clinical process that depends heavily on the judgment of the surgeon. Although some evaluation occurs before retrieval (ie chest radiographs and ICU bronchoscopy), most of the evaluation leading to the decision of utilization occurs at the time of organ retrieval. EVLP provides a more objective assessment of the lungs in an optimized environment, which is additionally important in DCDs, in which lung assessment in vivo is generally limited. Injury, as represented by the development of pulmonary edema during EVLP, is reflected in changes in compliance, airway pressure, PVR, and perfusate Po_2.[25] Despite Po_2 being one of the most important parameters during donor assessment in vivo, perfusate Po_2 is a less sensitive marker of lung injury during ex vivo evaluation, whereas dynamic compliance was the most sensitive functional parameter of pulmonary edema development.[26] Although Steen[14] originally proposed a single assessment after rewarming of the organ, we strongly believe that functional parameters should be monitored carefully and EVLP allowed to proceed over a period of at least 3 to 4 hours before any decision of organ utilization. Thus, trends during the procedure are more informative and at least stability of function is required for organ acceptance. We have generally used an EVLP delta Po_2 (pulmonary vein pO_2 minus pulmonary artery Po_2) of 400 mm Hg (on a fraction of inspired oxygen of 100%) as a cutoff value for lung acceptance for transplantation.[27] In addition to functional assessments, sequential lung

radiographs, flexible bronchoscopies, and lung deflation tests (by disconnecting endotracheal tube from the ventilator) can also provide valuable information during EVLP.

Using the EVLP assessment strategy described earlier, a clinical trial was performed by the Toronto Lung Transplant Program (HELP trial) using EVLP for the assessment of high-risk lungs that otherwise would not be used.[27,28] Eighty percent of the lungs that originally did not meet acceptance criteria from both BDDs and DCDs were ultimately transplanted after EVLP and resulted in posttransplantation outcomes equivalent to those of contemporary standard controls. Rates of PGD 3 at 72 hours after transplantation, need for extracorporeal membrane oxygenation, and airway complications have been extremely low (less than 5%). This experience has now been extended to more than 100 clinical lung transplants in Toronto with a 5-year survival rate of 70% in this population compared with 63% in contemporaneous transplants. EVLP transplants currently account for about 20% to 30% of our lung transplant activities and in 2013 was the major variable responsible for a 28% increase in our lung transplant activities. The routine or selective use of EVLP for DCD lung evaluation is still controversial. Good results have been achieved with the DCD LTx without EVLP[2,29] and further studies are required to determine the best strategy to expand DCD lung practices.

ASSESSMENT OF DONOR LUNGS USING BIOMARKERS DURING EX VIVO LUNG PERFUSION

Use of biological markers in lung tissue, in bronchoalveolar lavage, and in perfusate could significantly enhance determination of organ quality and predictability of transplant outcomes. In the past decade, several biomarkers have been explored

Table 1
Prospective clinical trials with EVLP

Name	Sponsor	Location	Method	Donor Type	Portable	Status
HELP	Vitrolife	Toronto	Toronto	Extended	No	Completed
NOVEL	XVIVO	United States	Toronto	Extended	No	Completed
INSPIRE	Transmedics	Europe/United States	OCS	Standard[a]	Yes	Recruiting
EXPAND	Transmedics	Europe/United States	OCS	Extended	Yes	Recruiting
DEVELOP	Vivoline	United Kingdom	Steen	Extended	No	Recruiting
Vienna	XVIVO	Vienna	Toronto	Standard[a]	No	Recruiting
Perfusix	Perfusix	United States	Toronto	Extended	LPC	Recruiting

Abbreviations: HELP, Human Ex Vivo Lung Perfusion; LPC, lung perfusion center.
[a] Randomized.

as important markers of donor lung injury. Cytokines such as interleukin (IL)-8, IL-1β, and IL-6 seem to reflect injuries on different levels, and IL-10 was shown to be protective.[16,30–32] Other studies have shown that biochemical markers such as endothelial nitric oxide synthase and cyclic guanosine monophosphate during EVLP may predict acceptable allograft function.[33] In contrast, a traditional injury marker such as lactate has failed to show a correlation with allograft acceptance or outcomes after transplantation.[34] Many other important markers have been discovered using high-throughput analyses such as microarrays and metabolomics.[35–37] EVLP will greatly enhance the capability to bring biomarker assessment to a real-time test in the clinical arena. Technology development to perform these diagnostic tests in a few hours rather than a few days is a parallel need, and this field continues to evolve.[38,39]

SYSTEMS AND TECHNIQUES FOR EX VIVO LUNG PERFUSION

Although in many places the current system in use is the one described in Toronto,[28] commercially available platforms for EVLP are now in various stages of development and approvals. Among them are the XPS system by XVIVO Perfusion, the LS1 by Vivoline Medical, and the Organ Care System by Transmedics. These systems of EVLP have some fundamental differences that have recently been described in detail.[3,40]

STATIC VERSUS MOBILE EX VIVO LUNG PERFUSION

The assumption that cold ischemia is detrimental to the donor lung underlies the development of mobile normothermic perfusion such as the OCS Lung system.[41] However, it remains unproved that limited cold ischemia is detrimental in the EVLP context. To date, no experimental evidence supports that periods of cold ischemia of several hours before and/or after EVLP lead to deleterious effects after transplantation. Mulloy and colleagues[42] showed added benefit of 4 hours of static cold preservation time before EVLP compared with normothermic EVLP without any cold ischemia. Our group has recently shown both in large animals and humans that long periods of CIT before or after EVLP does not have an adverse impact in recipient outcomes. We also think that cold preservation clinically provides a necessary margin of safety during the period of surgical implantation in which the warm atelectatic state could be injurious to the donor lung. Although the results of the INSPIRE trial may show equivalence or a benefit to recipients receiving standard criteria donor lungs that underwent machine perfusion during transportation versus cold ischemia alone, this does not answer whether the minimization of cold ischemic times before EVLP had any impact on observed patient outcomes.

A different randomized study also using standard criteria lungs is currently underway in Vienna using the Toronto method, in which no minimization of the first cold ischemic time will occur (stationary system). This study will help to further clarify this question. It is very likely that the intervention of normothermic EVLP at some point during the total preservation period is the major driver of donor lung quality improvement that is being observed in many studies. Thus, compelling experimental and clinical data showing that continuous, mobile, normothermic perfusion is superior to a combination of intervals of cold ischemic preservation and normothermic evaluation and treatment are needed to justify the conversion to this strategy considering the logistical challenges and the added expense needed for mobile normothermic perfusion of standard criteria lungs.

TREATMENT STRATEGIES

Rather than aiming solely at minimizing cold ischemia and improving lung evaluation, normothermic preservation instead has great promise for treating and rehabilitating injured donor lungs. This concept is transformative in clinical LTx; to be able to improve donor lungs rather than just preserve them in the condition in which they are found. Given that most potential donor lungs are injured by a variety of mechanisms including brain death, contusion, aspiration, infection, edema, and atelectasis, it could be envisioned that targeted therapies for each of these injuries could be delivered ex vivo for repair to significantly increase the donor lung pool.[3] The potential treatment opportunities and strategies during EVLP are shown in **Fig. 1**. Preclinical studies with the use of EVLP for lung repair have recently been reported. Each of these studies targeted a different form of donor lung injury and it is this breadth of exploration that will ultimately result in an arsenal of ex vivo lung therapy techniques applicable to each uniquely injured donor lung. This process will lead to transplant clinicians being able to apply a personalized medicine approach to the management of each donor lung. Pulmonary edema is a common injury seen in donor lungs secondary to brain death physiology and/or ICU fluid management before

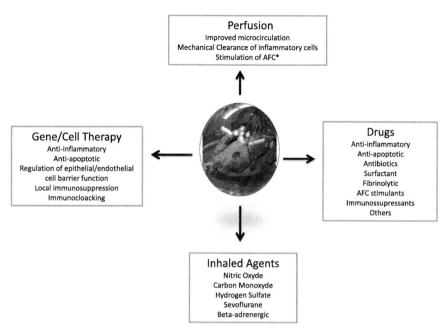

Fig. 1. Treatment strategies during normothermic EVLP.

retrieval. The use of terbutaline has been shown to accelerate the clearance of alveolar fluid during perfusion.[43] Another common mechanism of injury is aspiration. Inci and colleagues[44] attempted to improve porcine lungs injured by acid aspiration. By lavaging the donor lung with surfactant during EVLP, they were able to achieve improved graft function compared with controls. Because of the significant number of lungs rejected for suspicion of infection or pneumonia, delivery of high doses of antibiotics during EVLP is attractive. Both the Newcastle and Toronto groups have early data showing potential reduction in the burden of infection following EVLP antimicrobial therapy applied to infected human donor lungs.[45,46] We recently demonstrated the use of histopathologic analysis plus tissue plasminogen activator for diagnosis confirmation and therapeutic ex vivo thrombolysis of donor lungs affected with significant amounts of blood clots. The recipient receiving those lungs had an excellent outcome.[47]

EVLP-based gene and cellular therapy have also been explored. Ex vivo gene therapy with an adenoviral vector is effective and additionally attractive because of reduced vector-associated inflammation. Furthermore, this strategy can easily fit into the logistical flow of clinical LTx, simplifying clinical translation and adoption.[48] We have shown that EVLP-based IL-10 gene therapy for rejected human donor lungs results in improved function and reduced biomarkers of inflammation,

suggesting that IL-10 gene therapy could possibly increase the resilience of all donor lungs to reperfusion.[24] Lee and colleagues[49] have shown that the delivery of mesenchymal stem cells to EVLP lungs can restore endothelial barrier permeability and alveolar fluid balance after endotoxin-induced lung injury.

EX VIVO LUNG PERFUSION AS A BIOREACTOR FOR LUNG REGENERATION

Recent work from Ott and colleagues[50] and Petersen and colleagues[51] has shown a significant advance in lung regeneration. To regenerate gas exchange tissue, they seeded decellularized scaffolds from rat lungs with epithelial and endothelial cells. To establish function, they perfused and ventilated cell-seeded constructs in a bioreactor simulating the physiologic environment of a developing lung. By day 5, constructs could be perfused with blood and ventilated using physiologic pressures, and they generated gas exchange comparable with that of isolated native lungs. Transplanted lungs performed gas exchange for up to 6 hours. Although the methods described are only an initial step toward the long-term goal of generating functional lung tissue, the demonstration of a regenerated implantable organ that was able to maintain separation between the blood and airway compartments and that could participate in gas exchange for a period of time is very promising.

SUMMARY

Key advances in lung preservation in the form of hypothermia, inflated storage, and low-potassium dextran flush have culminated in the maturation of LTx into a standard of care for end-stage lung disease around the world. The emphasis of lung preservation is now shifting from hypothermic slowing of organ death to facilitating organ recovery and regeneration before implantation using normothermic EVLP technology. It is hoped that development of an ex vivo treatment arsenal ranging in complexity from pharmacologic to gene and cellular therapies will one day allow clinicians to use the full potential of the donor organ pool to engineer superior donor organs to improve the outcomes of LTx.

REFERENCES

1. Punch JD, Hayes DH, LaPorte FB, et al. Organ donation and utilization in the United States, 1996–2005. Am J Transplant 2007;7:1327–38.
2. Wigfield CH, Love RB. Donation after cardiac death lung transplantation outcomes. Curr Opin Organ Transplant 2011;16:462–8.
3. Munshi L, Keshavjee S, Cypel M. Donor management and lung preservation for lung transplantation. Lancet Respir Med 2013;1:318–28.
4. De Meester J, Smits J, Persijn G, et al. Listing for lung transplantation: life expectancy and transplant effect, stratified by type of end-stage lung disease, the Eurotransplant experience. J Heart Lung Transplant 2001;20:518–24.
5. Lederer DJ, Arcasoy SM, Wilt JS, et al. Six-minute-walk distance predicts waiting list survival in idiopathic pulmonary fibrosis. Am J Respir Crit Care Med 2006;174:659–64.
6. Hopkinson DN, Bhabra MS, Hooper TL. Pulmonary graft preservation: a worldwide survey of current clinical practice. J Heart Lung Transplant 1998;17: 525–31.
7. Fischer S, Matte-Martyn A, De Perrot M, et al. Low-potassium dextran preservation solution improves lung function after human lung transplantation. J Thorac Cardiovasc Surg 2001;121:594–6.
8. Southard JH, Belzer FO. Organ preservation. Annu Rev Med 1995;46:235.
9. Muller C, Hoffmann H, Bittmann I, et al. Hypothermic storage alone in lung preservation for transplantation: a metabolic, light microscopic, and functional analysis after 18 hours of preservation. Transplantation 1997;63:625–30.
10. Pegg DE. Organ preservation. Surg Clin North Am 1986;66(3):617–32.
11. Carrel A, Lindbergh CA. The culture of whole organs. Science 1935;81:621–3.
12. Jirsch DW, Fisk RL, Couves CM. Ex vivo evaluation of stored lungs. Ann Thorac Surg 1970;10:163–8.
13. Steen S, Sjoberg T, Pierre L, et al. Transplantation of lungs from a non-heart-beating donor. Lancet 2001; 357:825–9.
14. Steen S, Liao Q, Wierup PN, et al. Transplantation of lungs from non-heart-beating donors after functional assessment ex vivo. Ann Thorac Surg 2003;76:244–52 [discussion: 252].
15. Steen S, Ingemansson R, Eriksson L, et al. First human transplantation of a nonacceptable donor lung after reconditioning ex vivo. Ann Thorac Surg 2007;83:2191–4.
16. Rega FR, Vanaudenaerde BM, Wuyts WA, et al. IL-1beta in bronchial lavage fluid is a non-invasive marker that predicts the viability of the pulmonary graft from the non-heart-beating donor. J Heart Lung Transplant 2003;24:20–8.
17. Rega FR, Jannis NC, Verleden GM, et al. Long-term preservation with interim evaluation of lungs from a non-heart-beating donor after a warm ischemic interval of 90 minutes. Ann Surg 2003;238:782–92.
18. Aitchinson JD, Orr HE, Flecknell PA, et al. Functional assessment of non-heart-beating donor lungs: prediction of post-transplant function. Eur J Cardiothorac Surg 2001;20:187–94.
19. Erasmus ME, Fernhout MH, Elstrodt JM, et al. Normothermic ex vivo lung perfusion of non-heart-beating donor lungs in pigs: from pretransplant function analysis towards a 6-h machine preservation. Transpl Int 2006;19:589–93.
20. Cypel M, Yeung JC, Hirayama S, et al. Technique for prolonged normothermic ex vivo lung perfusion. J Heart Lung Transplant 2008;27:1319–25.
21. Petak F, Habre W, Hantos Z, et al. Effects of pulmonary vascular pressures and flow on airway and parenchymal mechanics in isolated rat lungs. J Appl Physiol (1985) 2002;92:169–78.
22. Broccard AF, Vannay C, Feihl F, et al. Impact of low pulmonary vascular pressure on ventilator-induced lung injury. Crit Care Med 2002;30:2183–90.
23. Cypel M, Rubacha M, Yeung J, et al. Normothermic ex vivo perfusion prevents lung injury compared to extended cold preservation for transplantation. Am J Transplant 2009;9:2262–9.
24. Cypel M, Liu M, Rubacha M, et al. Functional repair of human donor lungs by IL-10 gene therapy. Sci Transl Med 2009;1:4ra9.
25. Yeung JC, Koike T, Cypel M, et al. Airway pressure and compliance in the evaluation of donor lung injury during protective ex vivo lung perfusion in a porcine brain death model. J Heart Lung Transplant 2011;30:S143.
26. Yeung JC, Cypel M, Machuca TN, et al. Physiologic assessment of the ex vivo donor lung for transplantation. J Heart Lung Transplantant 2012; 31:1120–6.

27. Cypel M, Yeung JC, Machuca T, et al. Experience with the first 50 ex vivo lung perfusions in clinical transplantation. J Thorac Cardiovasc Surg 2012; 144(5):1200–6.

28. Cypel M, Yeung JC, Liu M, et al. Normothermic ex vivo lung perfusion in clinical lung transplantation. N Engl J Med 2011;364:1431–40.

29. Levvey BJ, Harkess M, Hopkins P, et al. Excellent clinical outcomes from a national donation-after-determination-of-cardiac-death lung transplant collaborative. Am J Transplantant 2012;12:2406–13.

30. Kaneda H, Waddell TK, de Perrot M, et al. Pre-implantation multiple cytokine mRNA expression analysis of donor lung grafts predicts survival after lung transplantation in humans. Am J Transplantant 2006; 6:544–51.

31. De Perrot M, Sekine Y, Fischer S, et al. Interleukin-8 release during early reperfusion predicts graft function in human lung transplantation. Am J Respir Crit Care Med 2002;165:211–5.

32. Fisher AJ, Donnelly SC, Hirani N, et al. Elevated levels of interleukin-8 in donor lungs is associated with early graft failure after lung transplantation. Am J Respir Crit Care Med 2001;163:259–65.

33. George TJ, Arnaoutakis GJ, Beaty CA, et al. A physiologic and biochemical profile of clinically rejected lungs on a normothermic ex vivo lung perfusion platform. J Surg Res 2013;183:75–83.

34. Koike T, Yeung JC, Cypel M, et al. Kinetics of lactate metabolism during acellular normothermic ex vivo lung perfusion. J Heart Lung Transplantant 2011; 30:1312–9.

35. Anraku M, Cameron MJ, Waddell TK, et al. Impact of human donor lung gene expression profiles on survival after lung transplantation: a case-control study. Am J Transplantant 2008;8(10):2140–8.

36. Kang CH, Anraku M, Cypel M, et al. Transcriptional signatures in donor lungs from donation after cardiac death vs after brain death: a functional pathway analysis. J Heart Lung Transplant 2010;30(3):289–98.

37. Ray M, Dharmarajan S, Freudenberg J, et al. Expression profiling of human donor lungs to understand primary graft dysfunction after lung transplantation. Am J Transplant 2007;7:2396–405.

38. Das J, Kelley SO. Protein detection using arrayed microsensor chips: tuning sensor footprint to achieve ultrasensitive readout of CA-125 in serum and whole blood. Anal Chem 2011;83:1167–72.

39. Bojko B, Gorynski K, Gomez-Rios GA, et al. Low invasive in vivo tissue sampling for monitoring biomarkers and drugs during surgery. Lab Invest 2014;94:586–94.

40. Van Raemdonck D, Neyrinck A, Cypel M, et al. Ex-vivo lung perfusion. Transpl Int 2014. [Epub ahead of print].

41. Warnecke G, Moradiellos J, Tudorache I, et al. Normothermic perfusion of donor lungs for preservation and assessment with the organ care system lung before bilateral transplantation: a pilot study of 12 patients. Lancet 2012;380:1851–8.

42. Mulloy DP, Stone ML, Crosby IK, et al. Ex vivo rehabilitation of non-heart-beating donor lungs in preclinical porcine model: delayed perfusion results in superior lung function. J Thorac Cardiovasc Surg 2012;144:1208–15.

43. Frank JA, Briot R, Lee JW, et al. Physiological and biochemical markers of alveolar epithelial barrier dysfunction in perfused human lungs. Am J Physiol Lung Cell Mol Physiol 2007;293:L52–9.

44. Inci I, Ampollini L, Arni S, et al. Ex vivo reconditioning of marginal donor lungs injured by acid aspiration. J Heart Lung Transplant 2008;27:1229–36.

45. Karamanou DM, Perry J, Walden HR, et al. The effect of ex-vivo perfusion on the microbiological profile of the donor lung. J Heart Lung Transplant 2010; 29:S94.

46. Bonato R, Machuca TN, Cypel M, et al. Ex vivo treatment of infection in human donor lungs. J Heart Lung Transplant 2012;31:S97–8.

47. Machuca TN, Hsin MK, Ott HC, et al. Injury-specific ex vivo treatment of the donor lung: pulmonary thrombolysis followed by successful lung transplantation. Am J Respir Crit Care Med 2013;188: 878–80.

48. Yeung JC, Wagnetz D, Cypel M, et al. Ex vivo adenoviral vector gene delivery results in decreased vector-associated inflammation pre- and post-lung transplantation in the pig. Mol Ther 2012;20:1204–11.

49. Lee JW, Fang X, Gupta N, et al. Allogeneic human mesenchymal stem cells for treatment of E. coli endotoxin-induced acute lung injury in the ex vivo perfused human lung. Proc Natl Acad Sci U S A 2009;106:16357–62.

50. Ott HC, Clippinger B, Conrad C, et al. Regeneration and orthotopic transplantation of a bioartificial lung. Nat Med 2010;16:927–33.

51. Petersen TH, Calle EA, Zhao L, et al. Tissue-engineered lungs for in vivo implantation. Science 2010;329:538–41.

Expanding the Donor Pool
Donation After Cardiac Death

Haytham Elgharably, MD[a], Alexis E. Shafii, MD[b], David P. Mason, MD[b],*

KEYWORDS

• Lung transplantation • Donation after cardiac death • Ex vivo lung perfusion • Outcomes

KEY POINTS

• Donor shortage remains a limiting factor for expanding lung transplantation rates.
• Donation after cardiac death (DCD) has become a valuable approach to increase the donor pool.
• Outcomes of controlled DCD are promising and comparable to conventional lung transplantation.
• Ex vivo lung perfusion can be used to assess and improve the quality of injured grafts in uncontrolled DCD.

INTRODUCTION

Lung transplantation (LTx) represents a life-saving therapy for patients with end-stage lung disease. Since the first successful LTx, 50 years ago,[1] the number of patients listed for transplant has been steadily increasing. However, that increase has been constantly challenged by a donor shortage. Of the available organ donors, only 20% are typically acceptable for lung donation. Although the selection process may vary between institutions, there are common criteria for ideal donors, including age less than 55 years, history of smoking less than 20 years, less than 48 hours mechanical ventilation, Po_2 to Fio_2 greater than 300, and no evidence of infection or pulmonary edema.[2,3]

Over the last three decades, donation after brain death (DBD) constituted the primary source for LTx. Multiple approaches have been developed to overcome the supply-demand mismatch in LTx, such as living lobar donation, use of extended criteria donors, ex vivo lung perfusion (EVLP), and donation after cardiac death (DCD).[4–7] This article reviews DCD LTx and its value in increasing the LTx donor pool.

DONATION AFTER CARDIAC DEATH

The first human lung transplant was performed by Dr James Hardy at the University of Mississippi in 1963 using a DCD donor. Formal criteria for brain death had not yet been established. This patient survived briefly although several decades passed before successful outcomes were reported using DCD lung donors. In 1995, D'Alessandro and colleagues[8] reported the first successful LTx from a DCD donor. Planned withdrawal of life support was performed in the operating room using controlled conditions. The recipient was on extracorporeal membrane oxygenation for severe rejection following a recent LTx for end-stage chronic obstructive pulmonary disease. Four days after retransplantation, the patient was successfully weaned and extubated. Although the posttransplant course was complicated by rejection 81 days later, and the patient ultimately expired 3 months after retransplantation, this was generally considered to be a success in DCD LTx.

In 2001, Steen and colleagues[9] also reported successful transplantation of lungs retrieved from

The authors have nothing to disclose.
a Department of Thoracic and Cardiovascular Surgery, Cleveland Clinic, 9500 Euclid Avenue, Cleveland, OH 44195, USA; b Department of Thoracic Surgery and Lung Transplantation, Baylor University Medical Center, 3409 Worth Street, Suite 640, Dallas, TX 75246, USA
* Corresponding author.
E-mail address: David.Mason@Baylorhealth.edu

Thorac Surg Clin 25 (2015) 35–46
http://dx.doi.org/10.1016/j.thorsurg.2014.09.011
1547-4127/15/$ – see front matter © 2015 Elsevier Inc. All rights reserved.

a donor who suffered from an acute myocardial infarction and died after failed resuscitation efforts. Intrapleural cooling was applied 65 minutes after death to preserve the lungs, and, 3 hours later, the right lung was transplanted into a 54-year-old woman with end-stage chronic obstructive pulmonary disease. Follow-up at 5 months posttransplant demonstrated good graft function.[9] These initial cases set the stage for increased use of DCD lungs for transplantation. The use of DCD lungs has grown internationally with DCD lungs accounting for 2% of lung transplants in the United States, 5% in Canada, 4.4% in Europe, 13.3% in the United Kingdom, and 22.5% in Australia.[10]

Maastricht Classification

With the intent of expanding DCD use, the first international workshop for DCD was held in Maastricht in the Netherlands in 1995 to further characterize potential donors after cardiac death.[11] Four categories of donors were identified (**Table 1**). Category I (dead on arrival) and II (unsuccessful resuscitation) were considered to be uncontrolled donors, whereas category III (awaiting cardiac arrest) and IV (cardiac arrest in a brain-dead donor) were considered to be controlled donors.

The controlled DCD (cDCD) scenario entails withdrawal of life-support measures in the intensive care unit (ICU) or operating room. Benefits of DCD donation include the ability to allocate the organ in advance, relative ability to predict cardiac arrest, and opportunity to evaluate graft function. Furthermore, it permits time for family discussion and to obtain consent. Potential donors of uncontrolled DCD (uDCD) typically suffer from unexpected cardiac arrest and/or unsuccessful cardiopulmonary resuscitation. In these scenarios, evaluation of graft function a priori is not feasible. Additionally, it is often difficult to precisely identify the time interval between cessation of circulation and the start of organ preservation measures,

defined as the warm ischemia (WI) time. The duration of WI can directly affect graft function after transplantation. Accordingly, reliable assessment of organ function is necessary before procurement.[9] Considering the limitations of uDCD donors, Maastricht category III has been considered by LTx centers as the DCD donor of choice for expansion of the donor pool.[10,12–14] In some countries more recently, donation after euthanasia (medically assisted death) has become and accepted practice and is considered as cDCD analogous to Maastricht category III. Proper DCD classification is essential to compare outcomes after LTx.

Eligibility for Donation After Cardiac Death

Potential donors for cDCD are typically patients with irreversible cerebral injury, high spinal cord injury, or end-stage musculoskeletal disorders who are expected to die within 60 minutes following withdrawal of life-support.[15] An algorithm has been developed by The University of Wisconsin to predict the expiration of potential DCD donors based on the patient's cardiopulmonary status, age, body mass index, and need for vasopressors.[16] Similarly, The United Network for Organ Sharing has proposed cardiopulmonary criteria that have been found useful in identifying potential DCD donors.

DeVita and colleagues[17] validated these predictive models in 505 patients who died in the ICU at variable time points after withdrawal of life support. They suggested that additional criteria be added to the predictive model for the likelihood of donor expiration including Glasgow Coma Scale, Pao_2/Fio_2 ratio, and peak inspiratory pressure. Other models have been developed with the inclusion of neurologic criteria and hemodynamic parameters at the time of withdrawal of life support.[18] Use of these predictive tools has further improved the ability to define eligibility for lung donation in the DCD setting.

DONATION AFTER CARDIAC DEATH LUNG PROCUREMENT
Warm Ischemia

An important difference between the brain dead donor and the non-beating-heart donor is the additional WI interval. As defined by the American Society of Transplant Surgeons, total WI time is "the period between withdrawal of life-support and initiation of organ perfusion," and true WI time is "the time between significant organ hypoperfusion (mean arterial pressure <60 mm Hg) and initiation of organ perfusion."[19] WI in uDCD is the time between cessation of circulation and

Table 1		
Maastricht classification of DCD donors		
Category I	Dead on arrival	Uncontrolled
Category II	Unsuccessful resuscitation	Uncontrolled
Category III	Awaiting cardiac arrest After planned withdrawal of life support	Controlled
Category IV	Cardiac arrest in a brain dead donor	Controlled

initiation of organ preservation measures. In cDCD, WI is the interval between withdrawal of life support and the initiation of organ preservation. Different terminologies have been suggested in the literature to define and study the phases of WI (**Fig. 1**)[18,20]:

- Withdrawal phase: life-support withdrawal to circulatory arrest
- No-touch period: circulatory arrest to death declaration
- Warm to cold interval: death declaration to starting organ preservation (cold ischemia).

During the agonal phase, there is progressive hypoxemia and hypoperfusion before circulatory arrest. The length of the agonal phase varies among donors, resulting in gradations of ischemic organ injury. Oto and colleagues[21] suggested that the clinical parameters that most directly correlate with the commencement of WI and organ damage are an oxygen saturation below 85% or systolic arterial pressure less than 50 mm Hg. Importantly, the length of the agonal phase is strongly believed to affect posttransplant graft function.[22,23] Snell and colleagues[23] showed that longer WI times were associated with lower Pao_2/Fio_2 ratios 24 hours after lung transplant and longer ICU stays. For this reason, most DCD protocols limit the acceptable agonal phase to 60 minutes for consideration for lung donation.

In addition to the variable agonal phase in DCD, is the so-called no-touch period. However, this timeframe is debated both legally and ethically and customarily determined by local regulations of the donor hospital. Most no-touch periods range from 2 to 5 minutes, although they may be as long as 20 minutes.[19,24,25] Some DCD protocols include time intervals for topical cooling before instillation of intravascular preservation.

Heparinization

In the DCD setting, heparin is typically administrated before cardiac arrest. However, due to the possibility of accelerating death in patients with intracerebral hemorrhage, pre-arrest heparinization is not universally allowed in all donor hospitals. Concerns for thromboembolism in unheparinized DCD donors have resulted in some hesitations in accepting nonheparinized donors for lung procurement. Oto and colleagues[26] looked at the incidence of unexpected donor thromboembolism in a clinical series of 122 lung donors by examining retrograde effluent for the presence of thrombus. They found a 38% incidence of unexpected thromboembolism and correlated its presence with worse outcomes after transplant. In another series, the same group reported that unexpected donor thromboembolism significantly increased the chances for primary graft dysfunction (PGD) after LTx.[27]

In a canine model of DCD LTx, it was shown that heparinization after cessation of circulation was effective in preventing microthrombi formation in the donor lungs.[28] Heparin also proved effective in preventing pulmonary embolism when administered within 30 minutes following cardiac arrest.[29] Additionally, retrograde flush of the pulmonary veins seemed helpful in clearing clot in the allograft when heparin was administered in a delayed fashion.[30–32] Similar findings by other investigators have also demonstrated that delayed heparin administration after cardiac death does not seem to affect thrombus formation in a DCD model of lung procurement.[33–36] In response to local restrictions on pre-arrest heparinization, some transplant centers administer postmortem heparin, which is then circulated with chest compressions following the declaration of death.[9,22,23,37,38] Although it seems that DCD lungs can be safely used without prearrest heparinization, heparin is preferrred to minimize the risks of thromboembolism.[22]

Donation After Cardiac Death Lung Preservation Techniques

Organ preservation protocols aim to minimize the WI interval with most centers accepting less than 60 minutes.[20] Following declaration of death, organ preservation is performed expeditiously. In

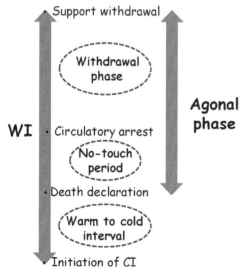

Fig. 1. Phases of WI in cDCD. CI, cold ischemia. (*Adapted from* Neyrick A, Van Raemdonck D, Monbaliu D. Donation after circulatory death: current status. Curr Opin Anesthesiol 2013;26:384; with permission.)

general, a hypothermia-based protocol is used that is similar to that used for DBD donors.

Cooling of the donor lungs can be achieved either topically or by cold antegrade perfusion of the pulmonary artery. Steen and colleagues[9] initially described techniques for rapid topical cooling. Many centers have adopted this technique.[37,39,40] An alternative is in situ cooling via continuous intrapleural infusion of Perfadex (4°C) via chest tubes[41] or directly on surgical exposure of the organs.[7] A potential advantage of in situ topical cooling is that it permits longer preservation of uncontrolled donors, allowing more time for family discussions and recipient allocation.[9,20]

Cold antegrade perfusion is still considered the gold standard method for organ preservation and defines the endpoint of WI. Following surgical exposure of the cadaveric lungs and venting of the left atrium, infusion of cold preservation solution via the pulmonary artery is performed to cool and flush the organs of remaining blood.[7,42] Perfadex (low potassium dextran solution) is the most commonly used preservation solution and is frequently supplemented with additional buffers and vasodilators.[7,10,43,44] Retrograde flush of the pulmonary veins is commonly performed to clear any remaining blood from the graft.[7]

Evaluation of Lungs for Donation After Cardiac Death

Assessment of lung function in DCD is a critical step in reducing the incidence of posttransplantation graft failure, especially considering the variability in WI time. Similar to methods used with brain dead donors, functional assessment of the donor lungs before cDCD can be achieved by bronchoscopy, chest radiography, arterial blood gases, and gross examination.[21,23,45] In the uDCD scenario, premortem functional evaluation is not possible. Accordingly, some method of that has been used is infusion of donor blood through the pulmonary artery and arterial blood gas assessment in the left atrium after arrest.[37,39,40] Alternatively, functional assessment can be carried out with by EVLP following organ retrieval.

Ex Vivo Lung Perfusion

The use of EVLP has gained popularity due to its ability to more accurately assess graft function before transplantation and potentially for its ability to improve organ function. Many consider EVLP to be a promising method for expanding the donor pool. With the growing acceptance of DCD lung usage, ex vivo perfusion is also being used to evaluate the suitability of DCD lungs for transplantation.

The development of EVLP has been pioneered by Steen and colleagues. Utilizing an extracorporeal circuit with adjustable perfusion and ventilation, lung function is able to be assessed ex-vivo and in some instances improved with variable durations of ex-vivo treatment. Perfusates that are used may be cellular (containing red blood cells) or acellular. Protocols typically target perfusion flow to 40% of the estimated donor cardiac output with maintenance of pulmonary artery pressures below 20 mm Hg to prevent lung injury.[46] The initial experience with EVLP was complicated by the development of pulmonary edema and deterioration of graft function[47] thought to be due to, hyperperfusion and the use of inappropriate pulmoplegia solutions.

Steen and colleagues[48] were the first to successfully apply EVLP. Key to the success was the development of Steen solution, a hyperosmolar perfusate that seemed to prevent pulmonary edema.[9,48] In an early case report, the investigators demonstrated excellent lung function from a donor with 50 minutes of unsuccessful resuscitation, 65 minutes of no-touch period, and 3 hours of intrapleural cooling. Subsequently, ex vivo evaluation of pulmonary allografts has been demonstrated by multiple investigators.[13,49–53] In 2006, Egan and colleagues[52] used EVLP to assess the function of human lungs that were deemed unsuitable for transplantation.[54] They reported improved oxygenation function after EVLP. Similarly, investigators at Lund University demonstrated that a prolonged period of EVLP can improve graft function.[55] The University of Toronto, group has also successfully performed EVLP for 12 hours in a porcine LTx model.[56,57]

From a clinical prospective, normothermic EVLP may prove to provide more benefits than static cold preservation. The Toronto group conducted a prospective study evaluating the use of ex vivo reconditioning in clinical LTx.[6] Out of 136 patients transplanted, lungs from 20 donors (9 DCD and 11 DBD) were identified as high risk for transplantation and were subjected to 4 hours of ELVP. No significant differences were found in 30-day mortality, ICU, or total hospital stay. The 1-year survival rate was 80% in the EVLP group and 83% in the control group ($P = .54$).[6]

Other LTx groups have also used EVLP to evaluate and recondition grafts that were initially rejected for LTx. In the United Kingdom, Zych and colleagues[58] reported their experience with 6 lungs that were initially rejected for transplantation and were then reconditioned for approximately 2 hours with EVLP (mean 141 ± 28.83 minutes). These were successfully transplanted with a

3-month survival of 100%. In Austria, Aigner and colleagues[59] were also able to improve the function of 9 out of 13 lungs turned down for transplant with EVLP and successfully utilized the lungs for transplantation. Currently, multicenter international trials are underway to better understand the value of EVLP in donor organ evaluation.

Ethical Considerations

Ethical considerations remain a major impediment to widespread acceptance of DCD. To minimize concerns regarding the donation process, conflicts of interest of health care providers that may affect decisions in care must be avoided. The decision to withdraw life-support should be discussed with the patient or family based on the futility of medical therapy. The foundation of ethical DCD practice is the "dead donor rule," which states that the death of a donor must be declared before organ retrieval can commence and that the retrieval process must not alter or hasten death.[60,61] To address these practical and ethical requirements, a no-touch period has been designated to confirm that death is permanent. In DCD protocols, the diagnosis of death is based on cardiopulmonary criteria, not neurologic criteria. This definition is "irreversible or permanent cessation of respiration and circulation."[15] The defined criteria are determined through absent heart sounds, absent pulse, and lack of spontaneous respiration. Intraarterial monitoring and Doppler interrogation are commonly used to document these findings.

One concern in DCD donor retreival is the phenomenon of autoresuscitation. This is defined as the spontaneous resumption of cardiopulmonary activity after circulatory arrest. To account for this possibility in DCD protocols and avoid organ procurement from a patient who may in fact return to life, the no-touch period has been established. This period must pass before organ procurement can commence. This no-touch period varies among hospitals, although is generally accepted to be between 2 and 5 minutes after loss of pulsatile circulation. According to an Organ Procurement Organization survey, most transplant centers in the United States apply a 5-minute no-touch period before declaration of death.[15] In some countries, the no-touch period can be extended up to 20 minutes.[25] A consensus opinion by the Society of Critical Care Medicine regarding the no-touch period recommended a minimum of 2 minutes and not more than 5 minutes of observation.[62]

Another ethical consideration with DCD is donation following physician-assisted suicide. Organs from these patients are presumed to behave similarly to cDCD and brain dead donors given the rapidity of their onset of death and short WI time. Regulations in this practice have been issued by some European countries (Netherlands, Belgium, and Luxembourg).[63,64]

EXPERIMENTAL DONATION AFTER CARDIAC DEATH LUNG TRANSPLANTATION
Feasibility of Lung Transplantation After Cardiac Death

Compared with other solid organs, the lung is unique in that does not solely depend on blood perfusion for cellular oxygenation. Passive diffusion of oxygen through the alveolar wall occurs directly into pulmonary epithelial cells for aerobic metabolism. As a result of this ability to maintain cellular viability by postmortem mechanical ventilation, the lung can tolerate extended intervals of circulatory arrest. Egan and colleagues[65] documented the extended viability of cadaveric lungs by maintaining postmortem ventilation in a canine model. Good graft function was maintained in the study at 1 hour of circulatory arrest although function began to decline when circulatory arrest was extended to 2 hours. Other investigators also documented the feasibility of DCD LTx in an experimental setting. Van Raemdonck and colleagues[66] reported lung tolerance to WI up to 1 hour, and Greco and colleagues[67] demonstrated successful LTx after WI intervals up to 90 minutes. Loehe and colleagues[68] similarly showed acceptable graft function after 90 minutes WI and 19 hours of cold storage.

One shortcoming of these experimental studies has been that the onset of cardiac death is abruptly induced and, therefore, does not reproduce the agonal phase of dying that occurs in the clinical setting of DCD procurement. Using a porcine model, Van de Wauwer and colleagues[69] observed significant sympathetic activation during the agonal phase of death with the subsequent development of pulmonary edema. Moreover, they determined that graft quality was affected by the pattern of cardiac death and that lung function was worse after extended periods of hypoxic arrest compared with rapid death induced by ventricular fibrillation or exsanguination. Similarly, in a rat model, premortem hypotension was shown to be associated with pulmonary edema and graft dysfunction.[70] As a result of the concerns raised by these experimental studies, most transplant centers limit the acceptable donor agonal phase to be 1 hour.

Donation After Cardiac Death Versus Donor After Brain Death Lung Transplantation: Brain Death–Induced Lung Injury

Brain death is known to cause a catecholamine surge that has been shown to induce neurogenic

Table 2
Clinical outcomes of donation after cardiac death lung transplantation

DCD LTx Series	WI	PGD	Acute Rejection	Airway Complications	Bronchiolitis Obliterans Syndrome	Survival
De Oliveira et al,[38] 1993–2009 Wisconsin (cDCD; n = 18)	30 ± 17 min	PGD 2/3: 33.3% DCD vs DBD: P = .59	A1, A2, A3: 27.8, 33.3, 0% DCD vs DBD: P = .03, .38, .39	DCD: 27.8% DBD: 12.8% P = .08	1, 3, 5 y: 19.6, 19.6, 27.7% DCD vs DBD: P = .59	1, 3, 5 y: 88.1, 81.9, 81.9% DCD vs DBD: P = .66
Zych et al,[13] 2007–2011 UK (cDCD; n = 26)	15 min	PGD 2: 24, 48, 72 h: 29, 38, 38% PGD 3: 24, 48, 72 h: 4, 4, 4% DCD vs DBD: P = NS	A1, A2, A3: 12, 8, 4% DCD vs DBD: P = NS	DCD: 7% DBD: 3% P = NS	2, 3, 4 y: 17.1, 17.1, 17.1% DCD vs DBD: P = NS	2, 3, 4 y: 81.7, 81.7, 81.7% DCD vs DBD: P = NS
Mason et al,[7] 2004–2011 Cleveland (cDCD; n = 32)	23 ± 14 min	PGD 2: 24, 48, 72 h: 3, 0, 0% PGD 3: 24, 48, 72 h: 3, 6, 6% DCD vs DBD: P = NS	UD	DCD: 22% DBD: 18% P = NS	2.3 y: 16% DCD vs DBD: P = NS	30 d, 1, 2, 3, 4 y: 97, 91, 91, 91, 71% DCD vs DBD: P = NS
De Vleeschauwer et al,[44] 2007–2010 Belgium (cDCD; n = 21)	15 min	PGD 2: 24, 48, 72 h: 35, 20, 5% PGD 3: 24, 48, 72 h: 25, 15, 10% DCD vs DBD: P = NS	A1, A2, A3: 14, 5, 0% B1, B2, B3: 14, 10, 5% DCD vs DBD: P = NS	UD	DCD: 14% DBD: 10% DCD vs DBD: P = NS	6 mo, 1, 3 y: 95, 95, 71% DCD vs DBD: P = NS

Study	Warm ischemic time	PGD	Acute rejection			Survival
Van De Wauwer et al,[12] 2005–2009 Netherlands (cDCD; n = 35)	29 min	PGD 1–3: 24, 48, 72 h: 42, 53, 50% DCD vs DBD: P = NS	DCD A2 5.7% DBD A1 2.6% DCD vs DBD: P = NS	UD	DCD: 6 mo, 1, 2 y: 3, 0, 13% DBD: 6 mo, 1, 2 y: 16, 15, 16% DCD vs DBD: P = .037 at 1 y	1, 2, 3, 4, 5 y: 91, 91, 85, 73, 73% DCD vs DBD: P = .53
Levvey et al,[10] 2006–2011 Australia (cDCD; n = 72)	35.2 ± 4.0 min	PGD 3: DCD 8.5% DBD 20%	UD	DCD 1.4%	DCD 7%	1, 5 y: DCD 97, 90% DBD 90, 61% DCD vs DBD: P = .04
Cypel et al,[22] 2006–2008 Toronto (cDCD; n = 10)	14–45 min	PGD 3: 10%	DCD A2 20%	DCD 10%	DCD 0%	30 d, 9 mo: 100, 90%
Puri et al,[78] 2003–2008 St Louis (cDCD; n = 11)	—	PGD 3 DCD 36% DBD 18%	DCD A1 9% DCD A3 9%	DCD 9%	DCD 27%	Perioperative, 18, 32 mo: 82, 64, 64%
Gomez-de-Antonio et al,[41] 2002–2009 Spain (uDCD; n = 29)	114 min	PGD 1: 17% PGD 2: 17% PGD 3: 38%	UD	None	1, 3, 5 y: 11, 35, 45%	Perioperative, 3 mo, 1, 2, 5 y: 83, 78, 68, 57, 51%

Abbreviations: NS, not significant; UD, undetermined.

pulmonary edema. Removed from this catecholamine surge, it has been proposed that DCD donor lungs may have better function than DBD. Supporting this hypothesis, DCD lungs have been shown experimentally to be less susceptible to ischemia-reperfusion injury than DBD lungs.[49] The exact underlying mechanism of brain death–induced lung injury is not completely clear although two mechanisms have been proposed. First, the sympathetic storm that accompanies brain death markedly increases the peripheral vascular resistance, resulting in increased left ventricle end-diastolic pressure, wedge pressure, and pulmonary capillary pressure.[71] Second, brain death induces a systemic inflammatory reaction by a surge of cytokines.[72] Activated proinflammatory cytokines are known mediators for the mechanisms of lung injury related to systemic inflammatory response. A similar mechanism of cytokine mediated lung injury has been proposed for the development of neurogenic pulmonary edema in brain dead donors.

In a recent study from the Toronto group, gene expression profiles of inflammatory mediators in lung biopsies were evaluated in DBD and DCD donors.[73] In pretransplant and postreperfusion samples, the levels of proinflammatory cytokines (interleukin [IL]-6, IL-8, IL-1, and IL-10) were higher in DBD compared with DCD samples. Moreover, microarray analysis of the lung biopsies demonstrated a marked increase in activation of inflammatory pathways in DBD donors.[73] In another clinical study by the Toronto group, it was shown that elevated levels of IL-8 and the IL-6/IL-10 ratio correlated with early graft dysfunction[74,75] and posttransplant 30-days mortality.[76] Similarly, Fisher and colleagues[77] found that elevated IL-8 levels in donor bronchoalveolar lavage were associated with graft dysfunction and early posttransplant mortality.

CLINICAL DONATION AFTER CARDIAC DEATH LUNG TRANSPLANTATION OUTCOMES

In 1963, Hardy and colleagues[1] performed the first successful human LTx using an allograft from an uDCD donor 30 minutes after unsuccessful resuscitation. Subsequently, the recipient died 18 days after transplant due to renal failure. Over the following two decades, several DCD LTx were performed but with poor long-term outcomes. As a result of these initial poor outcomes, a shift into DBD LTx was adopted by centers pursuing LTx at that time. Interest in DCD LTx was renewed with the experimental work of Egan and colleagues[65] in 1991 and the first successful cDCD LTx by D'Alessandro and colleagues[8] in 1995.

Since the revival of interest in DCD LTx, most studies of cDCD donors have demonstrated early and midterm outcomes comparable to DBD LTx (**Table 2**).[7,13,38] However, in one small case series, Puri and colleagues[78] reported that DCD LTx outcomes (36% mortality at 18 months) were inferior to DBD LTx and recommended cautious selection of DCD lungs. A growing international database of DCD LTx suggests comparable outcomes between DCD and DBD.

Early Graft Function

Considering the extended WI times associated with DCD donors, there were initial concerns for problematic PGD. Surprisingly, most of the reports with DCD lungs do not differ significantly from DBD in respect to PGD. Nevertheless, a trend toward increased early graft dysfunction (PGD grade 3) has been noted in some series although most show improvement within 72 hours posttransplant. The incidence of PGD3 was highest in the St Louis and Madrid series (36% & 38%, respectively) and was associated with more extracorporeal membrane oxygenation (ECMO) usage although this has not been shown in the experiences of other groups.

Airway Complications

In spite of the recent advances in the LTx surgical techniques, airway anastomotic complications continue to be a serious problem after LTx. Central airways depend on bronchial arterial perfusion and may more vulnerable to ischemia than the lung parenchyma. However, the incidence of airway complications after DCD LTx has not been shown to be significantly different from DBD in most of the reported series. The highest incidence of airway complications was reported in the Wisconsin series (27.8% DCD vs 12.8% of DBD) but this high incidence of airway complication has not been reported elsewhere.

Chronic Rejection

Bronchiolitis obliterans syndrome (BOS) is a progressive and irreversible obstructive process that affects the small airways after LTx leading to graft failure. The incidence of BOS reported in DCD LTx series is no worse than that for DBD LTx and, in fact, in the series from the Netherlands, BOS was more frequently observed in the DBD group compared with the DCD LTx group at 1-year follow-up ($P = .037$). Although most of the experience with DCD LTx reflects cDCD donors, there was a notably high incidence of BOS (45%) with the use of uDCD donors as reported by the Madrid group.

Survival

In most DCD LTx series, early term and midterm survival rates are comparable, if not better, than DBD LTx. In the largest reported series (n = 72), Levvey and colleagues[10] reported survival rates of 97% and 90% at 1 and 5 years. Similarly excellent survival rates were shown in Wisconsin, USA; United Kingdom; Cleveland, USA; Belgium; and the Netherlands.

Uncontrolled Donation After Cardiac Death Lung Transplantation Outcomes

The lung transplant group from Madrid, Spain, has reported the largest series of uDCD LTx.[41] However, they reported a high rate of grade 3 PGD (38%), which led to high perioperative mortality (17%). Recently, they have shown better outcomes for uDCD using EVLP to assess donor organs.[79]

SUMMARY

DCD LTx has become a valuable approach to expand the donor pool. The avoidance of inflammatory mediators resulting from brain death may prove to favor DCD LTx compared with DBD. Concerns regarding assessment of uDCD lungs before transplantation may be mitigated by EVLP. In the future, the introduction of novel pharmacologic or biologic therapies using EVLP may lead to improved graft function. Recent expansion of EVLP applications to include DCD graft evaluation is a growing approach in expanding the utilization of DCD lungs. The authors' experience with DCD LTx using standardized selection, procurement, and implantation techniques has been excellent. The International Society of Heart and Lung Transplantation has created a DCD registry that now serves as an important tool to assess the outcomes of DCD LTx. Education of transplant coordinators, physicians, and surgeons will be critical in expanding the usefulness of this promising source of donor organs.

REFERENCES

1. Hardy JD, Webb WR, Dalton ML Jr, et al. Lung Homotransplantation in Man. JAMA 1963;186:1065–74.
2. Meyers BF, Lynch J, Trulock EP, et al. Lung transplantation: a decade of experience. Ann Surg 1999;230(3):362–70 [discussion: 370–1].
3. Merlo C, Orens J. Selection of candidates for lung transplantation. Curr Opin Organ Transpl 2007;12: 749–84.
4. Bowdish ME, Barr ML, Schenkel FA, et al. A decade of living lobar lung transplantation: perioperative complications after 253 donor lobectomies. Am J Transplant 2004;4(8):1283–8.
5. Botha P, Trivedi D, Weir CJ, et al. Extended donor criteria in lung transplantation: impact on organ allocation. J Thorac Cardiovasc Surg 2006;131(5): 1154–60.
6. Cypel M, Yeung JC, Liu M, et al. Normothermic ex vivo lung perfusion in clinical lung transplantation. N Engl J Med 2011;364(15):1431–40.
7. Mason DP, Brown CR, Murthy SC, et al. Growing single-center experience with lung transplantation using donation after cardiac death. Ann Thorac Surg 2012;94(2):406–11 [discussion: 411–2].
8. D'Alessandro AM, Hoffmann RM, Knechtle SJ, et al. Successful extrarenal transplantation from non-heart-beating donors. Transplantation 1995;59(7): 977–82.
9. Steen S, Sjoberg T, Pierre L, et al. Transplantation of lungs from a non-heart-beating donor. Lancet 2001; 357(9259):825–9.
10. Levvey BJ, Harkess M, Hopkins P, et al. Excellent clinical outcomes from a national donation-after-determination-of-cardiac-death lung transplant collaborative. Am J Transplant 2012;12(9):2406–13.
11. Kootstra G, Daemen JH, Oomen AP. Categories of non-heart-beating donors. Transplant Proc 1995; 27(5):2893–4.
12. Van De Wauwer C, Verschuuren EA, van der Bij W, et al. The use of non-heart-beating lung donors category III can increase the donor pool. Eur J Cardiothorac Surg 2011;39(6):e175–80 [discussion: e180].
13. Zych B, Popov AF, Amrani M, et al. Lungs from donation after circulatory death donors: an alternative source to brain-dead donors? Midterm results at a single institution. Eur J Cardiothorac Surg 2012;42(3):542–9.
14. Levvey B. Excellent early results of Australian DCD lung transplantation. J Heart Lung Transplant 2010; 31(2):S63–4.
15. Bernat JL, D'Alessandro AM, Port FK, et al. Report of a National Conference on Donation after cardiac death. Am J Transplant 2006;6(2):281–91.
16. Lewis J, Peltier J, Nelson H, et al. Development of the University of Wisconsin donation after cardiac death evaluation tool. Prog Transplant 2003;13(4): 265–73.
17. DeVita MA, Brooks MM, Zawistowski C, et al. Donors after cardiac death: validation of identification criteria (DVIC) study for predictors of rapid death. Am J Transplant 2008;8(2):432–41.
18. Neyrinck A, Van Raemdonck D, Monbaliu D. Donation after circulatory death: current status. Curr Opin Anaesthesiol 2013;26(3):382–90.
19. Reich DJ, Mulligan DC, Abt PL, et al. ASTS recommended practice guidelines for controlled donation after cardiac death organ procurement and transplantation. Am J Transplant 2009;9(9):2004–11.

20. Oto T. Lung transplantation from donation after cardiac death (non-heart-beating) donors. Gen Thorac Cardiovasc Surg 2008;56(11):533–8.

21. Oto T, Levvey B, McEgan R, et al. A practical approach to clinical lung transplantation from a Maastricht Category III donor with cardiac death. J Heart Lung Transplant 2007;26(2):196–9.

22. Cypel M, Sato M, Yildirim E, et al. Initial experience with lung donation after cardiocirculatory death in Canada. J Heart Lung Transplant 2009;28(8):753–8.

23. Snell GI, Levvey BJ, Oto T, et al. Early lung transplantation success utilizing controlled donation after cardiac death donors. Am J Transplant 2008;8(6):1282–9.

24. Detry O, Le Dinh H, Noterdaeme T, et al. Categories of donation after cardiocirculatory death. Transplant Proc 2012;44(5):1189–95.

25. Geraci PM, Sepe V. Non-heart-beating organ donation in Italy. Minerva Anestesiol 2011;77(6):613–23.

26. Oto T, Rabinov M, Griffiths AP, et al. Unexpected donor pulmonary embolism affects early outcomes after lung transplantation: a major mechanism of primary graft failure? J Thorac Cardiovasc Surg 2005;130(5):1446.

27. Oto T, Excell L, Griffiths AP, et al. The implications of pulmonary embolism in a multiorgan donor for subsequent pulmonary, renal, and cardiac transplantation. J Heart Lung Transplant 2008;27(1):78–85.

28. Inokawa H, Date H, Okazaki M, et al. Effects of postmortem heparinization in canine lung transplantation with non-heart-beating donors. J Thorac Cardiovasc Surg 2005;129(2):429–34.

29. Okazaki M, Date H, Inokawa H, et al. Optimal time for post-mortem heparinization in canine lung transplantation with non-heart-beating donors. J Heart Lung Transplant 2006;25(4):454–60.

30. Akasaka S, Nishi H, Aoe M, et al. The effects of recombinant tissue-type plasminogen activator (rt-PA) on canine cadaver lung transplantation. Surg Today 1999;29(8):747–54.

31. Sugimoto R, Date H, Sugimoto S, et al. Post-mortem administration of urokinase in canine lung transplantation from non-heart-beating donors. J Heart Lung Transplant 2006;25(9):1148–53.

32. Hayama M, Date H, Oto T, et al. Improved lung function by means of retrograde flush in canine lung transplantation with non-heart-beating donors. J Thorac Cardiovasc Surg 2003;125(4):901–6.

33. Keshava HB, Farver CF, Brown CR, et al. Timing of heparin and thrombus formation in donor lungs after cardiac death. Thorac Cardiovasc Surg 2013;61(3):246–50.

34. Van De Wauwer C, Neyrinck AP, Geudens N, et al. Retrograde flush following warm ischemia in the non-heart-beating donor results in superior graft performance at reperfusion. J Surg Res 2009;154(1):118–25.

35. Sanchez PG, Bittle GJ, Williams K, et al. Ex vivo lung evaluation of prearrest heparinization in donation after cardiac death. Ann Surg 2013;257(3):534–41.

36. Brown CR, Shafii AE, Farver CF, et al. Pathologic correlates of heparin-free donation after cardiac death in lung transplantation. J Thorac Cardiovasc Surg 2013;145(5):e49–50.

37. de Antonio DG, Marcos R, Laporta R, et al. Results of clinical lung transplant from uncontrolled non-heart-beating donors. J Heart Lung Transplant 2007;26(5):529–34.

38. De Oliveira NC, Osaki S, Maloney JD, et al. Lung transplantation with donation after cardiac death donors: long-term follow-up in a single center. J Thorac Cardiovasc Surg 2010;139(5):1306–15.

39. Nunez JR, Varela A, del Rio F, et al. Bipulmonary transplants with lungs obtained from two non-heart-beating donors who died out of hospital. J Thorac Cardiovasc Surg 2004;127(1):297–9.

40. Gamez P, Cordoba M, Ussetti P, et al. Lung transplantation from out-of-hospital non-heart-beating lung donors. One-year experience and results. J Heart Lung Transplant 2005;24(8):1098–102.

41. Gomez-de-Antonio D, Campo-Canaveral JL, Crowley S, et al. Clinical lung transplantation from uncontrolled non-heart-beating donors revisited. J Heart Lung Transplant 2012;31(4):349–53.

42. Tierney A, Foster R, Ogella D. A perfusionist's role in lung transplant preservation. Perfusion 2004;19(6):351–7.

43. Fischer S, Matte-Martyn A, De Perrot M, et al. Low-potassium dextran preservation solution improves lung function after human lung transplantation. J Thorac Cardiovasc Surg 2001;121(3):594–6.

44. De Vleeschauwer SI, Wauters S, Dupont LJ, et al. Medium-term outcome after lung transplantation is comparable between brain-dead and cardiac-dead donors. J Heart Lung Transplant 2011;30(9):975–81.

45. Mason DP, Murthy SC, Gonzalez-Stawinski GV, et al. Early experience with lung transplantation using donors after cardiac death. J Heart Lung Transplant 2008;27(5):561–3.

46. Cypel M, Yeung JC, Keshavjee S. Novel approaches to expanding the lung donor pool: donation after cardiac death and ex vivo conditioning. Clin Chest Med 2011;32(2):233–44.

47. Hardesty RL, Griffith BP. Autoperfusion of the heart and lungs for preservation during distant procurement. J Thorac Cardiovasc Surg 1987;93(1):11–8.

48. Steen S, Liao Q, Wierup PN, et al. Transplantation of lungs from non-heart-beating donors after functional assessment ex vivo. Ann Thorac Surg 2003;76(1):244–52 [discussion: 252].

49. Neyrinck AP, Van De Wauwer C, Geudens N, et al. Comparative study of donor lung injury in

heart-beating versus non-heart-beating donors. Eur J Cardiothorac Surg 2006;30(4):628–36.

50. Rega FR, Vanaudenaerde BM, Wuyts WA, et al. IL-1beta in bronchial lavage fluid is a non-invasive marker that predicts the viability of the pulmonary graft from the non-heart-beating donor. J Heart Lung Transplant 2005;24(1):20–8.

51. Rega FR, Jannis NC, Verleden GM, et al. Long-term preservation with interim evaluation of lungs from a non-heart-beating donor after a warm ischemic interval of 90 minutes. Ann Surg 2003;238(6):782–92 [discussion: 792–3].

52. Egan TM, Haithcock JA, Nicotra WA, et al. Ex vivo evaluation of human lungs for transplant suitability. Ann Thorac Surg 2006;81(4):1205–13.

53. Snell GI, Oto T, Levvey B, et al. Evaluation of techniques for lung transplantation following donation after cardiac death. Ann Thorac Surg 2006;81(6): 2014–9.

54. Wierup P, Haraldsson A, Nilsson F, et al. Ex vivo evaluation of nonacceptable donor lungs. Ann Thorac Surg 2006;81(2):460–6.

55. Pierre L, Lindstedt S, Hlebowicz J, et al. Is it possible to further improve the function of pulmonary grafts by extending the duration of lung reconditioning using ex vivo lung perfusion? Perfusion 2013;28(4):322–7.

56. Cypel M, Yeung JC, Hirayama S, et al. Technique for prolonged normothermic ex vivo lung perfusion. J Heart Lung Transplant 2008;27(12):1319–25.

57. Cypel M, Rubacha M, Yeung J, et al. Normothermic ex vivo perfusion prevents lung injury compared to extended cold preservation for transplantation. Am J Transplant 2009;9(10):2262–9.

58. Zych B, Popov AF, Stavri G, et al. Early outcomes of bilateral sequential single lung transplantation after ex-vivo lung evaluation and reconditioning. J Heart Lung Transplant 2012;31(3):274–81.

59. Aigner C, Slama A, Hotzenecker K, et al. Clinical ex vivo lung perfusion—pushing the limits. Am J Transplant 2012;12(7):1839–47.

60. Youngner SJ, Arnold RM. Ethical, psychosocial, and public policy implications of procuring organs from non-heart-beating cadaver donors. JAMA 1993; 269(21):2769–74.

61. Robertson JA. The dead donor rule. Hastings Cent Rep 1999;29(6):6–14.

62. Ethics Committee, American College of Critical Care Medicine, Society of Critical Care Medicine. Recommendations for nonheartbeating organ donation. A position paper by the Ethics Committee, American College of Critical Care Medicine, Society of Critical Care Medicine. Crit Care Med 2001;29(9): 1826–31.

63. Detry O, Laureys S, Faymonville ME, et al. Organ donation after physician-assisted death. Transpl Int 2008;21(9):915.

64. Ysebaert D, Van Beeumen G, De Greef K, et al. Organ procurement after euthanasia: Belgian experience. Transplant Proc 2009;41(2):585–6.

65. Egan TM, Lambert CJ Jr, Reddick R, et al. A strategy to increase the donor pool: use of cadaver lungs for transplantation. Ann Thorac Surg 1991;52(5): 1113–20 [discussion: 1120–1].

66. Van Raemdonck DE, Jannis NC, De Leyn PR, et al. Warm ischemic tolerance in collapsed pulmonary grafts is limited to 1 hour. Ann Surg 1998;228(6): 788–96.

67. Greco R, Cordovilla G, Sanz E, et al. Warm ischemic time tolerance after ventilated non-heart-beating lung donation in piglets. Eur J Cardiothorac Surg 1998;14(3):319–25.

68. Loehe F, Mueller C, Annecke T, et al. Pulmonary graft function after long-term preservation of non-heart-beating donor lungs. Ann Thorac Surg 2000;69(5): 1556–62.

69. Van de Wauwer C, Neyrinck AP, Geudens N, et al. The mode of death in the non-heart-beating donor has an impact on lung graft quality. Eur J Cardiothorac Surg 2009;36(5):919–26.

70. Tremblay LN, Yamashiro T, DeCampos KN, et al. Effect of hypotension preceding death on the function of lungs from donors with nonbeating hearts. J Heart Lung Transplant 1996;15(3):260–8.

71. Novitzky D, Wicomb WN, Rose AG, et al. Pathophysiology of pulmonary edema following experimental brain death in the chacma baboon. Ann Thorac Surg 1987;43(3):288–94.

72. Avlonitis VS, Fisher AJ, Kirby JA, et al. Pulmonary transplantation: the role of brain death in donor lung injury. Transplantation 2003;75(12): 1928–33.

73. Kang CH, Anraku M, Cypel M, et al. Transcriptional signatures in donor lungs from donation after cardiac death vs after brain death: a functional pathway analysis. J Heart Lung Transplant 2011; 30(3):289–98.

74. De Perrot M, Sekine Y, Fischer S, et al. Interleukin-8 release during ischemia-reperfusion correlates with early graft function in human lung transplantation. J Heart Lung Transplant 2001;20(2):175–6.

75. De Perrot M, Sekine Y, Fischer S, et al. Interleukin-8 release during early reperfusion predicts graft function in human lung transplantation. Am J Respir Crit Care Med 2002;165(2):211–5.

76. Kaneda H, Waddell TK, de Perrot M, et al. Pre-implantation multiple cytokine mRNA expression analysis of donor lung grafts predicts survival after lung transplantation in humans. Am J Transplant 2006; 6(3):544–51.

77. Fisher AJ, Donnelly SC, Hirani N, et al. Elevated levels of interleukin-8 in donor lungs is associated with early graft failure after lung transplantation. Am J Respir Crit Care Med 2001;163(1):259–65.

78. Puri V, Scavuzzo M, Guthrie T, et al. Lung transplantation and donation after cardiac death: a single center experience. Ann Thorac Surg 2009;88(5):1609–14 [discussion: 1614–5].

79. Moradiellos FJ, Naranjo JM, Córdoba M, et al. Clinical lung transplantation after ex vivo evaluation of uncontrolled non heart-beating donors lungs: initial experience. J Heart Lung Transplant 2011;30(4):S38.

Single Versus Bilateral Lung Transplantation
Do Guidelines Exist?

Varun Puri, MD, MSCI*, G. Alexander Patterson, MD,
Bryan F. Meyers, MD, MPH

KEYWORDS

- Single lung transplantation • Double lung transplantation • Quality of life • Pulmonary fibrosis
- Emphysema

KEY POINTS

- Single or double lung transplantation is often performed for end-stage emphysema or pulmonary fibrosis.
- Single lung transplantation may maximize benefit to society by splitting the donor block.
- Double lung transplantation provides greater benefit to individual patients.

INTRODUCTION

Lung transplantation (LTx) has been accepted therapy for end-stage pulmonary disease for more than 2 decades. Lung transplant operations, unlike other solid organ transplants, are unique in that the donor block may be used for one recipient for a bilateral transplant or split to potentially benefit 2 patients with a single lung transplant each. The technical aspects of both operations have been well described and do not pose significant challenges.[1,2] Vocal proponents of both approaches cite benefits for each, but there remains a lack of high-quality evidence comparing the two approaches. In the absence of quality data to guide decisions, practice patterns remain largely institution or individual specific and disparate. This article examines the relative benefits and drawbacks of single versus bilateral LTx for specific lung diseases supplemented by a summary of the available evidence (**Tables 1** and **2**).

Bilateral transplant is the only acceptable transplant modality in patients with septic lung disease like cystic fibrosis or bronchiectasis because of concerns about contaminating the new lung with preexisting infection. Thus, this article excludes septic lung disease and accepts, for that population, the superiority of a bilateral operation. In addition, older patients with secondary pulmonary hypertension have anecdotally been considered preferentially for a bilateral transplant; however, Brown and colleagues[20] recently showed excellent short-term and intermediate outcomes in patients aged 65 years or older receiving a unilateral transplant. Otherwise, both single and bilateral transplants have been performed for other common indications including chronic obstructive pulmonary disease (COPD),[7] interstitial lung disease (ILD),[10] and primary pulmonary hypertension.[21] Single-center and registry-based studies have published comparative periprocedural, intermediate, and long-term outcomes after single and bilateral lung transplant[1,3,4,6,7,10–17,19,21,22]; however, no randomized trials or prospective, controlled studies have evaluated these two operations. In addition, the relative individual, societal, and

Grant support: NIH K07CA178120, K12CA167540-02 (Paul Calabresi Award), V. Puri.
Division of Cardiothoracic Surgery, Department of Surgery, Washington University School of Medicine, Campus Box 8234, 660 South Euclid Avenue, St Louis, MO 63110, USA
* Corresponding author.
E-mail address: puriv@wudosis.wustl.edu

Thorac Surg Clin 25 (2015) 47–54
http://dx.doi.org/10.1016/j.thorsurg.2014.09.007

Table 1
Gross evaluation of relative advantages of single lung transplant (SLT) and bilateral lung transplant (BLT) based on published literature

Outcome Parameter	Advantage SLT	Advantage BLT
Duration of operation	+	−
ICU and hospital stay	−	−
Early mortality	−	−
FEV$_1$ improvement with LTx	−	+
QOL measures	−	−
Freedom from BOS	−	+
Long-term survival	−	+
Relative cost-effectiveness (individual perspective)	−	+
Maximum societal benefit	+	−
High-risk recipient	−	+

Abbreviations: BOS, bronchiolitis obliterans syndrome; FEV$_1$, forced expiratory volume in 1 second; ICU, intensive care unit; QOL, quality of life.

economic implications of these approaches have been widely debated.[11,17]

EARLY OUTCOMES

Advocates of single LTx cite the simpler technical nature, the avoidance of a sternotomy, and the shorter duration of the procedure[22] as major advantages leading to improved immediate and perioperative outcomes. A registry database study of patients with ILD by Meyer and colleagues[10] noted that early (1-month) survival in recipients aged 30 to 49 years was significantly better with single lung transplant (SLT) than bilateral lung transplant (BLT) (early, 90.9% vs 77.1%). Survival was also significantly better with SLT than BLT at this early time point in those patients aged 50 to 59 years (early, 89.5% vs 81.7%).[10] In contrast, a smaller institutional study by Minambres and colleagues[22] showed that the 30-day survival was 81% in patients who underwent SLT, and 92% in patients who underwent BLT. Multivariable regression modeling to adjust for covariates and selection bias found that type of operation was not independently associated with short-term survival. Early experience at our center also showed no difference in 30-day mortality between recipients of SLT or BLT in a population of patients with

pulmonary fibrosis.[4] A registry database study by Meyer and colleagues,[7] evaluating patients with COPD, also found no difference in 30-day mortality between SLT and BLT in patients up to 60 years of age. They did note a higher 30-day survival for SLT versus BLT (93% vs 78%); however, the patient population is from the 1991 to 1997 time period, when arguably the BLT operation was still being learned and perfected. In contrast, Chang and colleagues[12] evaluated a single-institution database and noted a better 3-month survival with BLT compared with SLT, and confirmed their findings in a multivariate analysis.

Other investigators have also compared commonly accepted measures of early postoperative outcomes and found no major difference between SLT and BLT.[22] Minambres and colleagues[22] noted identical duration of postoperative ventilation (SLT, 32 hours; BLT, 29 hours) and intensive care unit stay (SLT, 7 days; BLT, 6 days) after these two operations at their institution. In another single-center study reporting on patients with pulmonary hypertension, the median duration of intubation for the SLT and BLT (7.5 vs 10 days, respectively), length of stay in the intensive care unit (10 vs 16 days), and hospital stay (32 vs 52 days) were not significantly different.[3] Although the differences in that study were not statistically significant, the small sample size could not exclude the possibility that clinically important differences existed despite the absence of a statistically significant difference.

FUNCTIONAL STATUS AND QUALITY OF LIFE

Spirometry, as measured by forced expiratory volume in 1 second (FEV$_1$) or FEV$_1$% predicted, is a key objective indicator of functional status in patients both before and after transplantation. Spirometry is strongly correlated with QOL in the lung transplant population.[11] Mason and colleagues[14] studied the relative impacts of SLT and BLT on FEV$_1$ at their institution. In 379 adult recipients, 6372 evaluations of postoperative FEV$_1$ and forced vital capacity (FVC) were analyzed using longitudinal temporal decomposition methods for repeated continuous measurements. FEV$_1$% predicted was better after BLT compared with SLT (65%, 58%, and 59% vs 51%, 43%, and 40% at 1, 3, and 5 years; $P = .3$). FVC measurements followed a similar pattern. In patients who had BLT, the posttransplant gains were more stable with fewer declines in FEV$_1$ compared with patients who had SLT, but FEV$_1$ measurements in patients after BLT did not reach double the values of SLT recipients. The differences in FEV$_1$ values between SLT and BLT were most pronounced in patients with COPD as the indication for transplantation. The investigators concluded that, "the advantage of spirometry values alone may not justify double lung transplantation."[14]

Despite a growing interest in medical economics and patient-reported outcomes, health-related QOL has been infrequently assessed after LTx. Anyanwu and colleagues[8] used the EuroQol, a generic questionnaire developed to provide a simple method for assigning utility values to health, and for evaluating QOL after SLT, BLT, and heart-lung transplantation. Eighty seven patients awaiting LTx and 255 transplant recipients were enrolled. In the waiting list group, 61% reported extreme problems in at least 1 of the 5 EuroQol QOL domains compared with 20% SLT recipients and 4% BLT recipients at 3 or more years after transplantation. The mean utility value (values range from zero for death to 1 for perfect health) for waiting list patients was 0.31, whereas it was 0.61 for SLT and 0.82 for BLT at 3 years after LTx. Problems in all 5 domains of EuroQol were more frequent in single-lung recipients. Assessment with a visual analog scale showed a similar trend. This study suggested that BLT leads to greater improvement in QOL compared with SLT, and that the benefits are durable.

In 2005, Gerbase and colleagues[11] compared a variety of measures including the 6-minute walk test, and QOL using the St George Respiratory Questionnaire (SGRQ) and a visual analog scale in 44 patients who had undergone SLT (n = 14) or BLT (n = 20). The SGRQ primarily studies 3 domains: respiratory symptoms, ability to perform routine activities, and impact of disease on daily life. Patients were followed for more than 2 years. Both single and bilateral transplant led to significant improvement in $FEV_1\%$ predicted and QOL compared with baseline pretransplant status. However, significantly lower spirometry values were observed in patients after SLT compared with patients after BLT over the long-term follow-up, with the difference being 20% lower at each time point over 4 years. In contrast with the spirometric data, the performance on the 6-minute walk test and scores on the SGRQ were not significantly different between recipients of single versus bilateral transplants. Despite poorer objective parameters of recovery of lung function, SLT recipients had long-term exercise tolerance and QOL that was comparable with those seen in patients who received BLT.

LONG-TERM SURVIVAL

Meyer and colleagues[7] were among the first to study SLT versus BLT using data from the United Network of Organ Sharing (UNOS) registry. They evaluated 2260 lung transplant recipients (1835 SLT, 425 BLT) with COPD who underwent surgery between 1991 and 1997. Survival rates at 30 days, 1 year, and 5 years for the patients aged less than 50 years were 93.6%, 80.2%, and 43.6%, respectively, for the patients with SLT, and 94.9%, 84.7%, and 68.2%, respectively, for the patients with BLT. For patients aged 50 to 60 years, survival rates were 93.5%, 79.4%, and 39.8% for the patients with SLT compared with 93.0%, 79.7%, and 60.5% for the patients with BLT. For those older than 60 years, 1-year SLT survival was 72.9% compared with 66.0% for the BLT group. Multivariate modeling, used to adjust for selection bias that might steer younger and fitter recipients to a bilateral procedure, confirmed a greater hazard for posttransplant mortality in patients aged 40 to 57 years who received SLT compared with BLT. The investigators concluded that SLT may offer acceptable early survival for recipients with end-stage COPD; however, long-term survival data favor the bilateral strategy until the recipients are approximately 60 years of age.[7]

In a related study in 2005, Meyer and colleagues[10] analyzed posttransplant outcomes in patients with pulmonary fibrosis, again using the UNOS database. The study included data from 821 patients (636 SLT, 185 BLT), aged 30 to 69 years, who were operated on between 1994 and 2000. In crude univariate analysis, early (1-month) and late (3-year) survival after SLT in recipients aged 30 to 49 years was better than with BLT (early, 90.9% vs 77.1%; late, 63.8% vs 46.2%, respectively). Unmatched early survival was also better with SLT than BLT at these time points in those patients aged 50 to 59 years. However, multivariate analysis and propensity score matching failed to show a statistical difference between survival after SLT and BLT, although a trend favoring SLT was observed. The investigators concluded that their study results could not support the apparent preferential use of BLT for younger patients with pulmonary fibrosis.

A subsequent analysis of UNOS registry patients was conducted in 2006 by Nwakanma and colleagues,[13] who analyzed 1656 initial LTx recipients, 60 years of age or older, who underwent operations from 1998 to 2004. For the 364 (28%) BLT and 1292 (78%) SLT recipients, long-term survival was not statistically different between the two groups in multivariate analysis or propensity score–matched analysis. Idiopathic pulmonary fibrosis and a donor tobacco history of more than 20 pack-years were significantly associated with increased mortality.

Table 2
Summary of evidence comparing SLT and BLT operations

Study	Study Design	Source of Information	Number of Patients	Indication for Transplantation	Key Findings	Potential for Bias	Quality of Evidence
Gammie et al,[3] 1998	Retrospective	University of Pittsburgh	57	Pulmonary hypertension	Similar survival after SLT or BLT	Yes	Low
Meyers et al,[4] 2000	Retrospective	Washington University	45	Pulmonary fibrosis	Similar survival after SLT and BLT	Yes	Low
Anyanwu et al,[5] 2000	Retrospective	UK Cardiothoracic Transplant Audit	405	All	Splitting lung blocks led to 1.8 extra survivors per donor block	Yes	Low
Force et al,[6] 2011	Retrospective	UNOS Thoracic Transplant Database	3860	Pulmonary fibrosis	Similar survival after BLT and SLT in multivariate and propensity-matched analyses	Yes	Low
Meyer et al,[7] 2001	Retrospective	UNOS Thoracic Transplant Database	2260	COPD	BLT leads to longer survival in recipients younger than 60 y	Yes	Low
Anyanwu et al,[8] 2001	Cross sectional questionnaire survey	Multiple centers in United Kingdom	255	All	QOL better after BLT	Yes	Low
Hadjiliadis et al,[9] 2002	Retrospective	Duke University	225	All	Reduced risk for BOS with BLT	Yes	Low
Anyanwu et al,[5] 2002	Statistical modeling	UK Cardiothoracic Transplant Audit	—	All	Cost per quality-adjusted life-year gained lower with BLT	Yes	Low

Study	Type	Data source	N	Population	Conclusion		Quality
Meyer et al,[10] 2005	Retrospective	UNOS Thoracic Transplant Database	821	Pulmonary fibrosis	SLT leads to longer survival in recipients younger than 60 y	Yes	Low
Gerbase et al,[11] 2005	Prospective	University of Geneva	44	All	Similar exercise tolerance and QOL after SLT and BLT	Yes	Low
Chang et al,[12] 2007	Retrospective	University of Michigan	339	All	Better survival with BLT	Yes	Low
Nwakanma et al,[13] 2007	Retrospective	UNOS Thoracic Transplant Database	1656	All, ≥60 y old	Similar survival for SLT and BLT	Yes	Low
Mason et al,[14] 2008	Retrospective	Cleveland Clinic	463	All	Spirometry weakly favors BLT more than SLT	Yes	Low
Thabut et al,[15] 2008	Retrospective	ISHLT registry	9883	COPD	BLT provided survival advantage, especially at <60 y of age	Yes	Low
Weiss et al,[16] 2009	Retrospective	UNOS Thoracic Transplant Database	1256	Pulmonary fibrosis	BLT superior to SLT in high-risk patients	Yes	Low
Neurohr et al,[17] 2010	Retrospective	Ludwig-Maximilians University, Munich	76	Pulmonary fibrosis	BLT provided functional and survival advantage	Yes	Low
Yusen et al,[18] 2013	Retrospective	ISHLT registry	43,428	All	Longer survival after BLT	Yes	Low
Black et al,[19] 2014	Retrospective	UNOS Thoracic Transplant Database	728	All	Patients with high LAS did better with BLT	Yes	Low

Abbreviations: COPD, chronic obstructive pulmonary disease; ISHLT, International Society for Heart and Lung Transplantation; LAS, lung allocation score; UNOS, United Network of Organ Sharing.

In 2008, Thabut and colleagues[15] reported on 9883 patients who underwent LTx for COPD between 1987 and 2007 and were enrolled in the registry of the International Society for Heart and Lung Transplantation. Median survival for the cohort receiving LTx for COPD was 5.0 years. The proportion of patients who underwent BLT increased over the study period from 21% to 56%. Median survival after BLT was longer than that after SLT (6.41 years vs 4.59 years). After adjusting for baseline differences between the two populations, BLT was still associated with longer survival compared with SLT (hazard ratio for death was 0.83 [0.78–0.92]). However, BLT did not confer a survival advantage compared with SLT for patients who were 60 years of age and older (hazard ratio, 0.95 [0.81–1.13]).

More recently, Force and colleagues[6] conducted a health services research study using the prospectively maintained database of the UNOS from 1987 to 2008, evaluating 3860 patients with idiopathic pulmonary fibrosis. Unadjusted analysis, comparing survival based solely on BLT versus SLT, showed a significant survival advantage for the BLT group, with a mean survival of 7.4 years for the SLT group and 8.3 years for the BLT group. However, multivariate and propensity score–matched analyses failed to show any survival advantage for BLT. One-year conditional survival, evaluating the overall survival of those who lived for at least 1 year after LTx, favored BLT (hazard ratio, 0.73; 95% confidence interval, 0.60–0.87). The investigators noted that significant risk factors for early death were recipient age more than 57 years and donor age more than 36 years. They concluded that, "BLT should be considered for younger patients with idiopathic pulmonary fibrosis and results may be optimized when younger donors are used."

Perhaps the most comprehensive view of long-term survival is provided by the annual report from the registry of the International Society for Heart and Lung Transplantation. The society published its 2013 report summarizing data from 1994 to 2011.[8] Adults who underwent LTx had a median survival of 5.6 years with unadjusted survival rates of 88% at 3 months, 79% at 1 year, 64% at 3 years, 53% at 5 years, and 31% at 10 years. Patients undergoing BLT had a higher overall median survival compared with those undergoing SLT (6.9 years vs 4.6 years). In addition, recipients of BLT who survived to 1 year after transplantation had a conditional median survival of 9.6 years, compared with 6.5 years for recipients of SLT. The registry database also noted an improved survival for transplants performed in the most recent era. Our institutional data also support a 5-year survival

rate advantage in favor of BLT versus SLT when LTx is performed for emphysema (66.7% vs 44.9%).[23]

OUTCOMES IN HIGH-RISK RECIPIENTS

Weiss and colleagues[16] evaluated the UNOS database for 1256 patients with pulmonary fibrosis who underwent LTx between 2005 and 2007. They divided the population into quartiles based on the lung allocation score (LAS). Patients in the highest LAS quartile were more likely to receive BLT than SLT (59.5% vs 38.4%). In patients with the highest LAS, BLT was associated with a 14.4% lower risk of mortality at 1 year. This survival benefit was confirmed on multivariable analysis (hazard ratio, 2.09; 95% confidence interval, 1.07–4.10) as well as in sensitivity analyses incorporating pulmonary hypertension. There were no differences in the 30-day or 90-day mortalities between SLT and BLT in any quartile on unadjusted or multivariable adjusted analysis.

With UNOS data suggesting an improved overall survival in bilateral recipients compared with SLT, the interaction between the LAS and type of transplant was further studied by Black.[19] The investigators evaluated 8778 patients from the UNOS Thoracic Transplant Database and used propensity matching to minimize other differences between the high-LAS and low-LAS groups and between single and double lung transplants in the high-LAS group. They reported on 8050 patients with LAS less than 75 and 728 with LAS greater than or equal to 75. Significantly shorter survival was seen in subjects with high LAS who received an SLT compared with those with high LAS who received a BLT (1-year survival 49% vs 57%). This survival difference was a much greater than that seen in the same comparison among the low-LAS patient population. The investigators commented that, "In the future, it will be important to determine whether there is an LAS cutoff point above which a single lung transplant should not be considered."

CHRONIC REJECTION

Neurohr and colleagues[17] analyzed their institutional LTx database and compared 46 SLT recipients with 30 BLT recipients. All patients underwent LTx for pulmonary fibrosis. On univariate and multivariate analysis, SLT was a predictor for development of bronchiolitis obliterans syndrome (BOS) greater than or equal to stage 1. Subgroup analysis revealed no statistically significant difference for BOS-free survival between BLT recipients with or without pulmonary hypertension. Although episodes of acute rejection were a risk factor for development of BOS, there was no difference in the incidence of acute rejection episodes between patients with SLT and BLT. In another institutional study with small sample size (n = 44), Gerbase and colleagues[11] similarly noted that SLT was associated with a greater risk of BOS at 24 months (relative risk, 2.86; 95% confidence interval, 1.22–6.67).

Hadjiliadis and colleagues[9] conducted a single-center study to evaluate the incidence BOS after LTx. BOS was diagnosed in 41.3% of the recipients (93 of 225 patients) at a median time since transplantation of 4.2 years. SLT was associated with higher rates of BOS compared with BLT (49.3% vs 31.7%, respectively). After controlling for other patient characteristics, the type of transplant remained a significant predictor of the time to the onset of BOS in a multivariable regression model. The authors' own institutional data also show a greater incidence of BOS in recipients of SLT compared with recipients of BLT.[23]

However, these findings are not consistent across all studies. Meyer and colleagues, [7] in a UNOS database analysis of 2260 LTx recipients with COPD, did not note any difference in the rate of development of BOS between SLT and BLT over a 3-year posttransplant follow-up period.

ECONOMIC EVALUATION AND SOCIETAL BENEFIT

The cost-effectiveness of LTx versus medical therapy was studied by Anyanwu and colleagues,[24] who also compared SLT and BLT in their analysis. They deduced that, over a theoretic 15-year period, LTx yielded mean benefits (relative to medical treatment) of 2.1 and 3.3 quality-adjusted life-years for SLT and BLT, respectively. Over the same duration, the average cost of medical care to those not receiving transplants was estimated at $73,564, compared with $176,640 and $180,528 for SLT and BLT, respectively. The estimated costs per quality-adjusted life-year gained were $48,241 for SLT and $32,803 for BLT. Sensitivity analysis revealed that benefits could be maximized by improving the QOL and reducing maintenance costs after transplantation.

The potential societal benefit from treating 2 patients with every donor lung block has also been systematically evaluated. Anyanwu and colleagues[5] studied lung donors from whom both lungs were used for transplant in the United Kingdom between April 1995 and December 1998 as reported to the UK Cardiothoracic Transplant Audit. Splitting of lung blocks resulted in an extra 0.8 survivors per donor block, 0.1 survivors

free from rejection, and 0.6 symptom-free survivors at 1 year, compared with transplantation into 1 recipient. However, the rate of use of the lung block from 1 donor for 2 SLTs is not uniform. Speicher and colleagues[25] queried the UNOS database for all SLTs performed from 1987 to 2011. They stratified donors into 2 groups: those donating both lungs and those donating only 1. The investigators reported 10,361 SLTs during this period, originating from 7232 unique donors. Of these donors, only 3129 (43.3%) had both lungs used. There was no significant increase in use over time. Rarer blood groups and smaller body surface area, among other predictors, were associated with nonuse of the second lung.

RECOMMENDATIONS

Over the last decade, the proportion of BLTs as a part of all LTx operations has been progressively increasing, whereas the number of SLT operations being performed annually is stable.[18] This trend likely reflects a general acceptance of some advantages of a bilateral transplant to the individual patient. However, because there is conflicting, low-quality evidence, a strong recommendation cannot be made favoring one operation more than the other when either is possible. Our institutional preference is to perform BLTs for most of our patients, but to consider SLT on an individual basis for older patients with COPD or ILD, particularly if there is a significant difference in the perfusion to the 2 native lungs.

FUTURE DIRECTIONS

Despite the lack of reliable evidence, there is almost no possibility of conducting a successful randomized trial to compare SLT and BLT in the appropriate patient population. It is anticipated that further analyses of registry data and statistical modeling studies will be important over the next several years in further elucidating the relative merits and demerits of SLT and BLT.

REFERENCES

1. Lau CL, Patterson GA. Technical considerations in lung transplantation. Chest Surg Clin N Am 2003; 13:463–83.
2. Puri V, Patterson GA. Adult lung transplantation: technical considerations. Semin Thorac Cardiovasc Surg 2008;20:152–64.
3. Gammie JS, Keenan RJ, Pham SM, et al. Single-versus double-lung transplantation for pulmonary hypertension. J Thorac Cardiovasc Surg 1998;115: 397–402 [discussion: 402–3].

4. Meyers BF, Lynch JP, Trulock EP, et al. Single versus bilateral lung transplantation for idiopathic pulmonary fibrosis: a ten-year institutional experience. J Thorac Cardiovasc Surg 2000;120:99–107.

5. Anyanwu AC, Rigers CA, Murday AJ. Does splitting the lung block into two single lungs equate to doubling the societal benefit from bilateral lung donors? Comparisons between two single versus one bilateral lung transplant. Transpl Int 2000;13:S201–2.

6. Force SD, Kilgo P, Neujahr DC, et al. Bilateral lung transplantation offers better long-term survival, compared with single-lung transplantation, for younger patients with idiopathic pulmonary fibrosis. Ann Thorac Surg 2011;91:244–9.

7. Meyer DM, Bennett LE, Novick RJ, et al. Single vs bilateral, sequential lung transplantation for end-stage emphysema: influence of recipient age on survival and secondary end-points. J Heart Lung Transplant 2001;20:935–41.

8. Anyanwu AC, McGuire A, Rogers CA, et al. Assessment of quality of life in lung transplantation using a simple generic tool. Thorax 2001;56:218–22.

9. Hadjiliadis D, Davis RD, Palmer SM. Is transplant operation important in determining posttransplant risk of bronchiolitis obliterans syndrome in lung transplant recipients? Chest 2002;122:1168–75.

10. Meyer DM, Edwards LB, Torres F, et al. Impact of recipient age and procedure type on survival after lung transplantation for pulmonary fibrosis. Ann Thorac Surg 2005;79:950–7 [discussion: 957–8].

11. Gerbase MW, Spiliopoulos A, Rochat T, et al. Health-related quality of life following single or bilateral lung transplantation: a 7-year comparison to functional outcome. Chest 2005;128:1371–8.

12. Chang AC, Chan KM, Lonigro RJ, et al. Surgical patient outcomes after the increased use of bilateral lung transplantation. J Thorac Cardiovasc Surg 2007;133:532–40.

13. Nwakanma LU, Simpkins CE, Williams JA, et al. Impact of bilateral versus single lung transplantation on survival in recipients 60 years of age and older: analysis of United Network for Organ Sharing database. J Thorac Cardiovasc Surg 2007;133:541–7.

14. Mason DP, Rajeswaran J, Murthy SC, et al. Spirometry after transplantation: how much better are two lungs than one? Ann Thorac Surg 2008;85:1193–201, 1201.e1–2.

15. Thabut G, Christie JD, Ravaud P, et al. Survival after bilateral versus single lung transplantation for patients with chronic obstructive pulmonary disease: a retrospective analysis of registry data. Lancet 2008;371:744–51.

16. Weiss ES, Allen JG, Merlo CA, et al. Survival after single versus bilateral lung transplantation for high-risk patients with pulmonary fibrosis. Ann Thorac Surg 2009;88:1616–25 [discussion: 1625–6].

17. Neurohr C, Huppmann P, Thum D, et al. Potential functional and survival benefit of double over single lung transplantation for selected patients with idiopathic pulmonary fibrosis. Transpl Int 2010;23:887–96.

18. Yusen RD, Christie JD, Edwards LB, et al. The Registry of the International Society for Heart and Lung Transplantation: Thirtieth Adult Lung and Heart-Lung Transplant Report–2013; focus theme: age. J Heart Lung Transplant 2013;32:965–78.

19. Black MC, Trivedi J, Schumer EM 2nd, et al. Double lung transplants have significantly improved survival compared with single lung transplants in high lung allocation score patients. Ann Thorac Surg 2014. [Epub ahead of print].

20. Brown CR, Mason DP, Pettersson GB, et al. Outcomes after single lung transplantation in older patients with secondary pulmonary arterial hypertension. J Heart Lung Transplant 2013;32:134–6.

21. Pasque MK, Trulock EP, Cooper JD, et al. Single lung transplantation for pulmonary hypertension. Single institution experience in 34 patients. Circulation 1995;92:2252–8.

22. Minambres E, Llorca J, Suberviola B, et al. Early outcome after single vs bilateral lung transplantation in older recipients. Transplant Proc 2008;40:3088–9.

23. Cassivi SD, Meyers BF, Battafarano RJ, et al. Thirteen-year experience in lung transplantation for emphysema. Ann Thorac Surg 2002;74:1663–9 [discussion: 1669–70].

24. Anyanwu AC, McGuire A, Rogers CA, et al. An economic evaluation of lung transplantation. J Thorac Cardiovasc Surg 2002;123:411–8 [discussion: 418–20].

25. Speicher PJ, Ganapathi AM, Englum BR, et al. Single lung transplantation in the United States; what happens to the other lung? Oral Presentation at the 34th Annual Meeting of the International Society for Heart and Lung Transplantation. San Diego (CA). April 10–13, 2014.

Airway Complications After Lung Transplantation

Michael Machuzak, MD[a],*, Jose F. Santacruz, MD[b],
Thomas Gildea, MD[a], Sudish C. Murthy, MD, PhD, FACS, FCCP[c]

KEYWORDS

- Lung transplant • Bronchoscopy • Bronchial stenosis • Airway dehiscence • Airway necrosis

KEY POINTS

- Airway necrosis has a broad spectrum, and mild forms are expected in the early time after transplant.
- Severe airway complications are later term events associated with infection, rejection, and persistent ischemia and necrosis.
- Bronchoscopy has a major role in the complex management and a wide array of techniques are used in maintaining airway patency.
- Airway stenting in lung transplant is an option of last resort and requires specific expertise and long-term management.

INTRODUCTION

Airway complications (AC) have had a significant impact on the morbidity and mortality in lung transplantation since the first human lung transplant in 1963. Early incidence of complications were exceedingly high at 60% to 80%, but improvement in many facets led complication rates to drop significantly into the 10% to 15% range with a related rate of mortality of 2% to 3%.[1–6]

AC have a variety of presentations and, although their treatments are often institution-dependent, they are all individualized to the type of AC (stenosis, dehiscence, and so on), timing, location, and severity. Although most early reports of AC dealt primarily with the anastomosis, complications distal to the suture line, such as the "vanishing bronchus syndrome," are now being noticed.[7]

AC can be grouped anatomically (anastomotic or distal to the anastomosis), descriptively (stricture, granulation tissue, infection, necrosis, dehiscence, and fistula formation), temporally (early or late), or by cause (ischemic, infectious, iatrogenic, or idiopathic). In addition to the associated mortality, patients with AC experience increased morbidity, most notably in quality of life. The number of procedures, repeated office visits, hospitalizations, and associated costs can all significantly affect one's satisfaction with lung transplant and, in some cases, minimize or completely negate benefits from this complicated undertaking.

The goals of this article include a brief description of the history of AC, transplant-specific anatomy, surgical techniques of lung transplantation, classification of AC, causes, management, and potential future directions for prevention and treatment.

The authors have nothing to disclose.
[a] Department of Pulmonary, Allergy and Critical Care Medicine, Respiratory Institute, Cleveland Clinic, 9500 Euclid Avenue, Cleveland, OH 44195, USA; [b] Pulmonary, Critical Care and Sleep Medicine Consultants, Houston Methodist, Houston, TX 77030, USA; [c] Department of Thoracic and Cardiovascular Surgery, Heart and Vascular Institute, Cleveland Clinic, Cleveland, OH 44195, USA
* Corresponding author. Respiratory Institute, Cleveland Clinic, 9500 Euclid Avenue, M2-141, Cleveland, OH 44195.
E-mail address: machuzm@ccf.org

Thorac Surg Clin 25 (2015) 55–75
http://dx.doi.org/10.1016/j.thorsurg.2014.09.008
1547-4127/15/$ – see front matter © 2015 Elsevier Inc. All rights reserved.

HISTORICAL BACKGROUND

James Hardy performed the first human lung transplantation at the University of Mississippi in 1963. The patient had lung cancer and died 18 days after the transplant due to renal failure.[8]

The first successful lung transplant occurred at the University of Toronto in 1983. Before it, multiple attempts were performed around the world without success; many of those cases had deficient healing of the bronchial anastomosis.[8]

In the early days of lung transplantation, AC were a significant source of morbidity and mortality, making AC the "Achilles heel" of lung transplantation short-term survival.[1–3,8,9]

With improved surgical techniques, new immunosuppressant regimens, and overall better medical management, survival has significantly improved over the years.[1,10]

ANATOMY

Lung transplantation patients have a unique situation compared with other solid organ recipients. Human lungs contain dual blood supplies, a pulmonary and a separate bronchial circulation (**Fig. 1**). Bronchial circulation is not re-established in standard lung transplantation and provides the blood supply to the major airways and supporting structures of the lungs. Previous anatomic studies have defined fairly consistent origins of the bronchial arteries. These vessels arise either as branches of the aorta or as intercostal arteries and travel through the hila, where small arterials enter into the muscular layer of the airway and eventually terminate in a plexus within the bronchial mucosa. This submucosal plexus gives rise to a collateral circulation between the pulmonary and bronchial vessels. Each proximal mainstem bronchus receives its primary blood supply through the bronchial circulation, although the pulmonary circulation can contribute via retrograde collaterals. Although the pulmonary circulation is re-established during the transplantation procedure, bronchial vessels are not. This feature places bronchial viability and anastomotic healing completely dependent on retrograde blood flow from the pulmonary to bronchial circulation. As one can imagine, this has the potential for perioperative ischemia jeopardizing the anastomosis and distal airways. The main carina and both proximal mainstem bronchi are supplied via the coronary collateral system arising from atrial branches at the left and right coronary arteries, possibly explaining why the proximal airways seem to suffer less ischemic injury (see **Fig. 1**).

INCIDENCE AND PREVALENCE

There is a wide range in the reported incidence of anastomotic complications in the lung transplant population. Reports of complication rates range

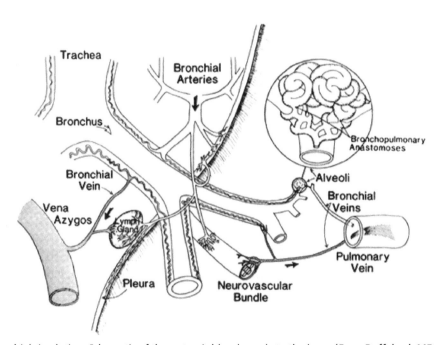

Fig. 1. Bronchial circulation. Schematic of the systemic blood supply to the lung. (*From* Deffebach ME, Charau NB, Lakshminarayan S, et al. State of the art: the bronchial circulation—small but vital attribute of the lung. Am Rev Respir Dis 1987;135:467; with permission.)

from 1.6% to 33% over the past several decades, although numbers around 15% seem to be the expert consensus. The incidence of AC in heart-lung transplant recipients is lower.[1,9,10] Many theories exist for the rationale of why AC rates have declined from the 60% to 80% range, including advances in graft preservation, donor and recipient selection, progress in perioperative management, including immunosuppression as well as enhancements in surgical techniques. Most recently, Shofer and colleagues[11] and Dutau and colleagues[12] reported institutional rates of AC of 13% and 14.5%, again on par with recent observations.[1–6,10,13–17] Controversy regarding the incidence of AC in transplantation using donations after cardiac death exists, but in the authors' experience, is similar to that reported for lung from brain-dead donors.[18,19]

This issue is clearly complex with much interplay, but one of the most likely reasons for this wide range may be the lack of a standardized classification system. What has been classified as a complication at one institution may not have been listed as one at another institution. AC classifications are discussed later in this article.

RISK FACTORS

Several proposed risk factors to the development of AC have been identified. These risk factors can be subdivided into donor/recipient factors, surgical techniques, infections, medications or immunosuppression, and miscellaneous.[20]

Historically, AC have been mainly attributed to ischemia of the donor bronchus during the immediate posttransplant period.[1,21,22]

DONOR AND RECIPIENT RISK FACTORS

Several risk factors may be attributed to the donor. Van De Wauwer and colleagues[9] identified the length of donor's mechanical ventilation (50–70 hours) before organ recovery and a greater height mismatch (likely related to a larger bronchial diameter) with a taller donor being more likely to lead to an AC.

In such cases, the surgical technique of minimizing the length of the anastomosis as well as telescoping may be the best solution.[10]

Other risk factors thought to be involved include ischemia of the donor bronchus (particularly in the immediate postoperative period), the length of the donor bronchus, the type of surgical anastomosis, infections, size difference between the donor and recipient bronchus, type of immunosuppressive regimen used, pulmonary fungal infections, and the need for a postoperative tracheostomy.[2,15,23–27]

SURGICAL

Which anastomotic technique is best is often debated, and there are certainly many theories as to which is superior.[10,28]

Many techniques and variations, including telescoping, end-to-end, wrapping vascular pedicels, and bronchial artery revascularization, have been tried and studied, and although opinions vary on which is best, no consensus is present. The initial experience of end-to-end anastomoses was poor, but fortunately, these outcomes prompted changes and led to a variety of techniques.[2,21]

After initial disappointing results, the practice of wrapping the anastomosis became more popular, first with omentum, later pericardial, peribronchial, or intercostal tissue.[2,4,25,26,28]

However, the added technical complexity of the wrap in addition to lack of randomized controlled trials showing benefit has decreased enthusiasm for this technique and it is rarely used today.[29]

The technique of telescoping the anastomosis has also been tried to address complications, particularly dehiscence.[2,17,22,30]

Although it initially gained support, this technique has been largely abandoned because it has demonstrated increased complication rates as high as 48%.[15]

The major issue limiting the usefulness of the telescoping technique was increased stenosis, but increased concern for infection has also been cited. These complications are likely related to this technique starting with a narrowed airway by virtue of the telescoping and possibly trapping bacteria between the airway walls.[10,15]

Presently, the end-to-end bronchial anastomosis without a wrap, performed as close to the secondary carina as possible, is the preferred technique at most centers.[10,31]

Performing the anastomosis close to the secondary carina is desirable, as donor bronchus length has been shown to be crucial. Excessive length of this donor bronchus increases the likelihood for ischemia because all flow in the posttransplant period is via collaterals and inversely proportional to length.[2,9,21]

Although it may seem logical that a longer ischemic time will increase the incidence of AC, this has not necessarily proven true and has been best supported in bilateral sequential lung transplantation.[3,8,14,17]

Despite the longer ischemic time, the second anastomosis of a bilateral sequential transplant is not more prone to AC.[25]

Regardless of the approach, the bronchial anastomosis remains ischemic in the postoperative period, possibly leading to AC. Bronchial artery revascularization (BAR) has been presented as an approach to avoid this and is discussed later.[10,17,26,28–32]

INFECTIONS

Infections in both the preoperative and the postoperative periods have long been postulated to be a factor predisposing to AC. The rationale of increased inflammation and decreased healing certainly has merit.[13,21]

In some patients, a high inoculum of pathogenic organisms may be present immediately after transplantation, and often the anastomosis is sutured on a contaminated field, not infrequently with multi-drug-resistant bacteria.[10,33,34]

Combining this with evidence supporting bacterial and fungal airway colonization, increasing patient risk for infections in suppurative lung disease, may add support[28,29,33,34]; however, the actual role of infection leading to dehiscence, stricture, granulation tissue, and malacia is not firmly established.

MEDICATIONS/IMMUNOSUPPRESSION

Considerable improvements in lung transplant survival have been achieved; however, other solid organ transplants demonstrate superior survival. Although AC may play a role, other factors contribute as well. Despite lung-transplant patients being maintained at higher levels of immunosuppression, both acute and chronic rejection rates remain higher than most solid organ transplants. Chronic rejection manifests as bronchiolitis obliterans syndrome (BOS) and occurs earlier with more dire consequences than other solid organ transplants.[35]

Immunosuppression is critical for the survival of an allograft; however, this may predispose to AC due to increased susceptibility to infection and diminished healing. The use of corticosteroids in the preoperative period was once considered a contraindication because of concern for anastomotic healing.[24,36]

Later studies showed not only adverse effect and possibly less granulation tissue formation but also improved survival in the face of corticosteroids.[2,25,36–38]

Typical posttransplant immunosuppressive regimens are 3-tiered and consist of a calcineurin inhibitor (typically tacrolimus), an antilymphocyte (mycophenolate mofetil or azathioprine), and a corticosteroid. Sirolimus (rapamycin, Rapamune) should specifically be discussed because it has been shown to play a role in airway healing. Sirolimus is a novel macrolide originally developed as an antifungal agent, later discovered to have potent immunosuppressive and anti-proliferative properties. Sirolimus was first used in renal transplants and later in lung transplants because the major complication associated with calcineurin inhibitors is renal toxicity, which is much less common with sirolimus. Sirolimus was shown to dramatically increase the rate of catastrophic AC in de novo recipients. In particular, the rate of dehiscence was found to be unacceptably high in the early transplant period. The current recommendation is avoidance of sirolimus for at least 90 days after transplantation.[24,27,39]

MISCELLANEOUS

Multiple other risk factors have been described as potential etiologic features for AC. These factors include primary graft dysfunction, acute cellular rejection, positive pressure mechanical ventilation, positive end-expiratory pressure (PEEP), organ preservation technique, recipient/donor sex or age, body mass index, and acute kidney injury, among others.[1,9,10,20,21,40–42]

Primary graft dysfunction, a type of reperfusion injury, may compromise pulmonary flow and increase the length of mechanical ventilation and the degree of PEEP required. Positive pressure mechanical ventilation and PEEP have the potential to increase the bronchial wall and the anastomosis stress, with the potential of inhibiting collateralization, and graft perfusion might be impaired when high inflation pressures are needed.[1,10]

Even though studies have described more AC with prolonged mechanical ventilation, controversy exists.[28]

Nevertheless, the literature varies from center to center and among periods of time; no consensus regarding the relationship of the above-mentioned miscellaneous risk factors to the development of AC has been achieved.

CLASSIFICATION OF AIRWAY COMPLICATIONS

AC are quite diverse and vary in presentation, severity, complexity, and timing. Bronchial stenosis is identified as the most common complication, but others should be included in the discussion, such as granulation tissue, malacia, infection, dehiscence, and fistula. Anastomotic complications, particularly early in the history of lung transplantation, played a major role in the less than optimal morbidity and mortality. Management of such problems can be complex and is best handled as a multidisciplinary team approach. Over the past decade, novel techniques have played a major role in the management of these complications. Balloon bronchoplasty, laser photoresection, electrocautery, high-dose-rate brachytherapy, cryotherapy, and stent placement among others have been described. Although there is little doubt these endoscopic techniques have played an important role, they certainly are not the only advancement in transplant medicine, as enhancements in medical management such as understanding graft dysfunction, immunologic reactions, antimicrobial prophylaxis as well as postoperative care have paved the way to improved outcomes.[1,6,17,21,22,43]

As previously mentioned, there is a wide range in the reported incidence of AC. One explanation may be the lack of a universal classification system. There have been several attempts at a classification system; however, none have been unanimously accepted.[2,24,44–46]

The authors have previously described the basic classification of AC.[1] The classification described the 6 types of AC with a brief description of the bronchoscopic, radiological, and clinical observations (**Box 1**; **Table 1**).

Box 1
Description of the macroscopic aspect, diameter, sutures (MDS) endoscopic standardized grading system for central airway complications after lung transplantation

M (macroscopic aspect)

M0: scar tissue

M1: protruding cartilage

M2: inflammation/granulomas

M3: ischemia/necrosis

- Extent of abnormalities in regard to the anastomosis

    a. Abnormalities localized to the anastomosis

    b. Abnormalities extending from the anastomosis to the bronchus intermedius or to the extremity of the left main bronchus, without lobar involvement

    c. Abnormalities extending from the anastomosis to lobar or segmental bronchi

    d. Abnormalities affecting the lobar and/or segmental bronchi, without anastomotic involvement

D (diameter)

D0: normal to a fixed reduction less than 33%

D1: expiratory reduction (malacia) greater than 50%

D2: fixed reduction from 33% to 66%

D3: fixed reduction greater than 66%

- Extent of abnormalities in regard to the anastomosis

    a. Abnormalities localized to the anastomosis

    b. Abnormalities extending from the anastomosis to the truncus intermedius or to the extremity of the left main bronchus, without lobar involvement

    c. Abnormalities extending from the anastomosis to lobar or segmental bronchi

    d. Abnormalities affecting the lobar and/or segmental bronchi, without anastomotic involvement

S (sutures)

S0: absence of dehiscence

S1: limited dehiscence (<25% of circumference)

S2: extensive dehiscence (from 25% to 50%)

S3: very extensive dehiscence (>50%)

- Localization: e: anteriorly; f: other localizations

From Dutau H, Vandemoortele T, Laroumagne S, et al. A new endoscopic standardized grading system for macroscopic central airway complications following lung transplantation: the MDS classification. Eur J Cardiothorac Surg 2014;45(2):e33–8; with permission.

Table 1
Description of airway complications after lung transplantation

Classification of Airway Complications	
Stenosis/ stricture	Anastomotic bronchial stenosis • Stenosis <50% of bronchial diameter • Stenosis >50% of bronchial diameter Nonanastomotic bronchial stenosis • Stenosis <50% of bronchial diameter • Stenosis >50% of bronchial diameter
Necrosis and dehiscence	Grade I • No slough or necrosis • Well-healed anastomosis Grade II • Any necrotic mucosal slough observed but no bronchial wall necrosis Grade III • Bronchial wall necrosis within 2 cm of anastomosis Grade IV • Extensive bronchial wall necrosis extending >2 cm from anastomosis
Exophytic granulation tissue	• Obstructing <50% of the bronchial lumen • Obstructing >50% of the bronchial lumen
Malacia	• Diffuse tracheal/bronchial • Anastomotic location
Fistula	• Bronchomediastinal fístula • Bronchopleural fístula • Bronchovascular fistula
Infectious	Anastomotic infections • Bacterial • Fungal Nonanastomotic infections • Bacterial • Fungal • Viral

Adapted from Santacruz JF, Mehta AC. Airway complications and management after lung transplantation: ischemia, dehiscence, and stenosis. Proc Am Thorac Soc 2009;6(1):79–93.

Recently, Dutau and colleagues[12] published a proposed grading system for central AC following lung transplantation; this is known as the MDS classification. The first parameter the system describes is the macroscopic aspect (M); the next described is the diameter (D), and a third describes the appearance of the sutures (S).

In the MDS classification system, the M designation is divided into 4 subgroups: M0, or the healed scar aspect, is considered by most to represent the normal response of healing; M1 (cartilaginous protrusion) is most commonly present in cases of size mismatch from the donor to recipient bronchi and is typically associated with a telescoping anastomosis, although there may be no abnormal healing and the lumen is narrowed simply due to the diameter of the donor bronchus; M2 (granulomatous component) is related to exuberant inflammation at the anastomotic site; and the M3 lesion describes ulceration, ischemia, and necrosis.

The D classifications are divided into 4 subgroups classifying the diameter: the D parameter is separated by the amount of reduction with D0, including a normal to fixed reduction up to 33%; D1, including malacia greater than 50%; D2, including a stenosis from 33% to 66%, and D3, including any stenosis greater than 66%.

The S designation was developed to include dehiscence ranging from S0 or absence of dehiscence to limited dehiscence of less than 25%; S2 categorizing dehiscence from 25% to 50%; and S3 extensive dehiscence greater than 50%.

It is the hope of these authors that a nomenclature and classification system will be universally accepted. This universal classification system may be the first step to scientifically approaching this morbid complication. Until issues such as AC can be consistently reported, its incidence, prevalence, morbidity, and mortality cannot be fully understood and consistent techniques for treatment and possibly prevention cannot be developed.

BRONCHIAL STENOSIS

Bronchial stenosis is the most common complication, with published reports between 1.6% and 32%.[13,15,47,48]

Extensive necrosis and dehiscence will predispose to the formation of strictures. Infectious causes may play a role as well, and *Aspergillus* has been identified as one potential causative agent. As discussed, the surgical technique may predispose an airway to stenosis with a 7% incidence seen in a telescoping anastomotic technique.[4,15] Recently, an association between early rejection and the incidence of strictures was described.[49]

Another important distinction when discussing bronchial stenosis is the location. The most commonly discussed bronchial stenosis involves a stricture at the anastomotic line; however, recent publications have highlighted another troubling finding of stenosis distal to the anastomotic line. This nonanastomotic stenosis can be quite troubling because the strictures can extend segmentally and even subsegmentally. This incidence is lower, although with the caveat that in many publications this type of stricture was not specifically labeled separately, so the reported rates of 2.5% to 3% may be inaccurate.[3,48,50]

This type of stricture can be severe enough to cause the loss of a segmental or larger airway, as in the case of the vanishing bronchus intermedius syndrome (VBIS) (**Fig. 2**). The bronchus intermedius may be particularly susceptible likely because it is already a narrower airway. This symptomatic narrowing occurs in approximately 2% of the airways. The most devastating form can lead to a complete atresia. VBIS can be seen as early as 6 months and adversely affects survival with a mean survival of 25 months after initial diagnosis.[7,50]

The underlying cause of bronchial stenosis is poorly understood but may be related to increased airway inflammation and a mononuclear infiltration. Coupled with ischemic injury, this can lead to changes in the underlying cartilage, epithelium, and re-formation of airway vessels.[3,37] Stenosis is typically seen 2 to 9 months posttransplant.[3,25,47,51]

Bronchial strictures may present asymptomatically and be diagnosed on routine posttransplant bronchoscopic surveillance, as early stenosis may have minimal clinical signs or symptoms. More frequently, it manifests as increasing dyspnea, cough, postobstructive pneumonia, radiographic abnormalities, or dropping flow rate on spirometry.[6]

The pulmonary function tests may show in spirometry a decrease in the forced and peak expiratory flow. Also, a spirometry failure to improve the in the first few months after transplant may be seen.[2] Abnormal flow-volume loops patterns have been described.[52,53]

Flexible bronchoscopy is the gold standard for diagnosis. CT of the chest is also useful in the diagnosis and for intervention planning. Axial, helical, and multiplanar reconstruction CT chest-imaging techniques have been described to have an accuracy of more than 90% in the diagnosis of bronchial stenosis.[54,55]

Multiple individual techniques have been described, although a multimodality approach is most common. Successful techniques are in continuous evolution but the armamentarium typically includes a multitiered approach with dilation, ablation, and stent placement in ascending order depending on the severity. Dilation can be accomplished by many means with an endoscopic balloon, a rigid scope, or a bougie. Ablation modalities are also numerous, with cryotherapy, electrocautery, laser, argon plasma coagulation (APC), brachytherapy, or even photodynamic therapy being described. Stenting should be left as a last resort, because although beneficial in many ways, stenting is not without potentially serious complications.[2,6,13,56–59]

Dilation is usually the first therapeutic procedure performed and can be accomplished safely in multiple ways, as in discussed later. Balloon bronchoplasty is the most common procedure and has been shown to be an excellent palliative technique, improving spirometry and relieving symptoms immediately in 50% and 94% of patients, respectively.[47] Although more than one procedure is typical, balloon bronchoplasty may be the only procedure required in 26% of cases.[56]

No single method has proven superiority, but personal experiences have shown several potential advantages with the inflatable balloon. These balloons come in a variety of sizes, allowing for incremental and customized dilations. Balloon dilation can also be done quickly and safely, often under conscious sedation without the need for fluoroscopy.[56,58] The procedural aspects have been well described previously and vary from device to device and so are beyond the scope of this article (**Fig. 3**).[47,60]

Balloon bronchoplasty is a simple and quick task to change a balloon size rather than upsizing rigid bronchoscopes for dilation, although it is more costly.

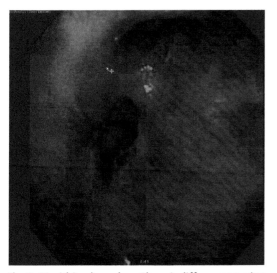

Fig. 2. Vanishing bronchus. There is diffuse narrowing of the graft but a notable stenosis of the bronchus intermedius disproportionate to the anastomosis and right upper lobe narrowing.

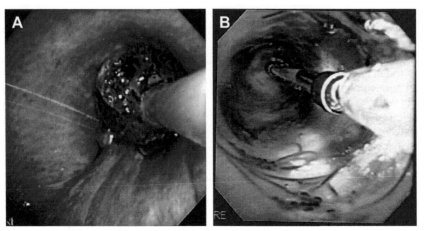

Fig. 3. (A) Balloon dilation across anastomosis. (B) Note the excessive suture and knots indicate healing dehiscence as the knots are supposed to be extraluminal.

The rigid bronchoscopic technique has advantages other than cost, because it allows for direct visualization during dilation, tissue debulking, and tamponade while simultaneously ventilating one or both lungs. An inflated balloon will completely occlude the airway it is dilating, preventing ventilation, and can be an issue when dealing with a single-lung transplant or a tracheal lesion (less commonly). An additional benefit of the rigid bronchoscope includes ease of stent placement, particularly if a silicone stent is being placed. Although rigid dilation is effective, care must be taken to avoid injury, endobronchial or otherwise, and should only be done by an experienced operator.[61,62]

Strictures can assume many shapes; some are focal and weblike, and others are dense and long. The type of stricture encountered will dictate the intervention. A focal weblike stricture may be best handled with a mucosal-sparing technique, such as electrosurgery or laser, followed by dilation.[63]

Adjunctive techniques, such as submucosal steroid injection or mitomycin-C, have also been described. In a technique adapted from published articles describing endoscopic treatment of tuberculosis strictures, small volumes of dexamethasone or a similar steroid are injected submucosally at the area of the stricture.[64] Although no controlled trial evidence exists for this technique, it has been described in lung-transplant patients as well.[63]

In a similar fashion, borrowing an idea from ENT literature, endobronchial mitomycin-C has also been described.[65]

Stenting may be required in cases of recurrent stenosis, although in this immune-compromised population, placement of any foreign body must be carefully considered. Historically, self-expanding metallic stents (SEMS) have been described more commonly in transplant patients. Published use of SEMS in anastomotic and postanastomotic stenosis can provide almost immediate relief in 80% to 94% of individuals as well as "long-term" maintenance of patency in 45% of patients.[47,66]

Despite the reported success in these patients, numerous complications have been described. Complications are not uncommon in any nonmalignant condition, particularly in a complex group of immune-compromised patients. The types and rates of complications vary and include infections (16%–33%), granulation tissue formation (12%–36%), and stent migration (5%).[6,66] This list is not all-inclusive because bacterial colonization, halitosis, and fatigue-related stent fracture are also well described. The halitosis may be related to bacterial colonization and bio-film formation within the stent. Colonization is seen in up to 78% of patients.[6,66,67] Although not all colonization is significant or needs to be treated, emerging data in stented patients may suggest that stents increase respiratory infections. Although this data come from patients with malignant airway disease, care must be taken in those immunosuppressed to the level of transplant patients.[68]

One must also keep in mind that once an SEMS is deployed, the next thought should be on removal. The longer an SEMS is in place, the more difficult it may be to remove, and the removal process can be quite complicated.[69–71] Fernandez-Bussy and colleagues[72] used completely covered SEMS to successfully treat transplant-related AC and described the potential removal in experience hands.

Stent-related complication rates as high as 54% are reported in transplant patients. This rate echoes concerns for stent placement in any benign disease.[73–75]

Although many experts think silicone stents are the preferred types of stents in benign diseases, particularly transplant airways, SEMS may have some advantages. Their ease of deployment, especially without a rigid bronchoscope, favorable external to internal diameter ratio, and superior flexibility allowing the stent to conform to the abnormalities associated with anastomoses can make them particularly useful.[76]

Given many concerns associated with SEMS, particularly in benign airway disease, silicone stents are gaining popularity. Many features of silicone stents make them ideal for lung transplant AC, including lower rates of granulation tissue, ability to be modified, and the ease of removal. The ability to customize these stents cannot be overestimated, because the exact length can be cut; customized holes can be fashioned to allow ventilation and mucus clearance from airways that would otherwise be compromised from a fully covered SEMS.[46,76,77] Stenting of the bronchus intermedius may be challenging because of the probable occlusion of the right upper lobe; in such case a customized silicone stent or a modified Montgomery T-tube should be used.[78] Sundset and colleagues[79] reported the successful use of silicone stents for stenotic AC, and that, after removal, the airways remained patent and had an improved spirometry value for as long as 24 months.

Silicone stents are not without complications, including increased rates of migration and mucus plugging, reinforcing that the decision to place any kind of stent must be carefully evaluated.[23]

Hybrid stents exist as well and have been described in transplant patients. The self-expanding silicone stent, Polyflex (Boston Scientific, Boston, MA, USA), is one example. The authors' experience with this was reported. They found this stent suboptimal, with a 100% migration rate, and have since abandoned its use in their practice.[75]

Regardless of the type of stent used, there can be complications, and one must be cognizant of this fact. No stent is perfect, and multiple authors have previously published the advantages and disadvantages.[74,75,80]

Presently, the authors' practice is to reserve the use of any stent only after other techniques have been exhausted, particularly in patients with recalcitrant symptomatic bronchial strictures in whom repeated balloon dilations have failed (**Fig. 4**).

Dutau and colleagues[81] retrospectively evaluated the clinical efficacy and safety of silicone stents in lung-transplant patients. They described the insertion of 17 silicone stents in 117 patients over a range of 5 to 360 days to palliate 23 airways. Symptomatic improvement was seen in all, with an increase in mean forced expiratory volume in 1 second (FEV1) of 672 ± 496 mL. The stent-related complication rate was 0.13 per patient per month, with obstructive granulomas (10), mucus plugging (7), and migration (7) being the most common. Stents were successfully removed in 16 of 23 airways and the stented patients had a similar survival to those without AC.

An area of interest related to the significance of AC specifically is stenosis. Castleberry and colleagues[49] looked at risk factors and outcomes of bronchial stricture because they may be associated with acute rejection. A total of 9335 patients were analyzed with a stricture incidence of 11.5%. They found that early rejection was associated with a significantly greater incidence of strictures. Also associated with increased incidence of stricture were male gender, restrictive lung disease, and pretransplant requirement of hospitalization. Those with a stricture had a lower postoperative peak percent predicted FEV1, shorter unadjusted survival, and an increased risk of death after adjusting for potential confounders.

In a single-center retrospective review, Shofer and colleagues[11] evaluated lung-transplant patients with central airway stenosis (CAS) with the objective of determining its association with chronic rejection or worse survival. Also, risk factors associated with CAS were identified. In this review, 467 patients were evaluated with 60 (13%) developing CAS. Of the patients with CAS, 22 (37%) had resolution with bronchoplasty alone; 32% required stent. This retrospective review determined that CAS requiring intervention was not a risk factor for developing BOS or worse survival, although it was a significant complication. Pulmonary fungal infections and the need for postoperative tracheostomy were identified as risk factors for the development of CAS based on their time-dependent multivariable model.

The multimodality approaches discussed have been shown to be effective, safe, and reproducible over time but are not infallible. When endoscopic techniques fail, a surgical approach can be considered. Bronchial anastomoses reconstruction, sleeve resections, bronchoplasty, lobectomy, pneumonectomy, and even retransplantation have all been described. As one can imagine, this comes at a cost of morbidity and mortality.

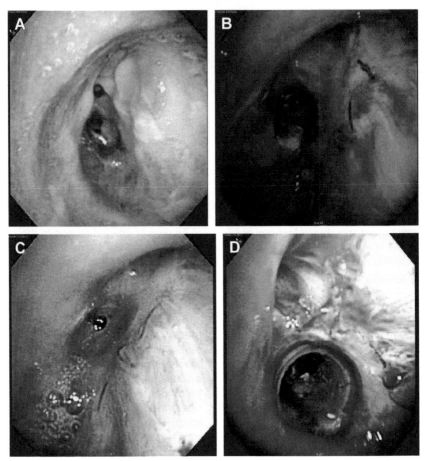

Fig. 4. Evolution of necrosis. (*A*) Development of necrosis and subsequent stricture formation. (*B*) Response to balloon bronchoplasty, with improvement in necrosis and diameter of lumen. (*C*) Recurrence of stricture, refractory to intermittent balloon bronchoplasty. (*D*) Eventual solution to stricture with silicone stent placement.

NECROSIS AND DEHISCENCE

Whether isolated at the anastomotic line or extending from it, some necrosis is seen almost universally after transplant. Because this finding is so common, it is often not referred to as a complication, but rather as part of the normal healing process. Necrotic changes are typically seen early in the healing process characteristically between weeks 1 and 5. The necrotic area is often circumferential, originating at the anastomosis, and can extend into lobar or even segmental bronchi (**Fig. 5**). This finding peaks early on and resolves quickly in most cases because the airway will either heal or progress to frank dehiscence. Bronchial necrosis and subsequent dehiscence can thus be viewed as a continuum from the normal to the catastrophic (**Fig. 6**).[10,82]

Although necrosis is commonplace, dehiscence is seen much less often with commonly reported incidences between 1% and 10%,[83] although a single report describes this finding in as many as 24% of airways, again likely owing to the variance in reporting.[15]

Although much is still not known of the inciting events leading to necrosis and dehiscence, it is likely that ischemia and infection play major roles in the most severe cases. Significant morbidity and mortality can be attributed to a frankly dehiscing airway. This devastating complication may still arise despite the most meticulous surgical techniques and uneventful postoperative course. A key to preventing the disastrous event may be early diagnosis, and this is best realized by always considering the diagnosis.

Early diagnosis is particularly important in any lung-transplant patient with a prolonged air leak, pneumothorax, or pneumomediastinum. Overt dehiscence can be difficult to diagnose because many of the signs or symptoms of dehiscence are commonly seen in the posttransplant period, attributed to other more common complications. A chest roentgenogram is crude but may intimate dehiscence by a pneumothorax or pneumomediastinum,

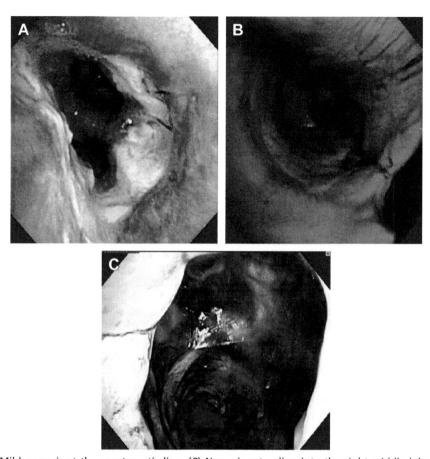

Fig. 5. (*A*) Mild necrosis at the anastomotic line. (*B*) Necrosis extending into the right middle lobe. (*C*) Severe necrosis with continued ischemia.

whereas a chest CT has a higher degree of sensitivity and specificity.[84]

A CT scan may show dehiscence as evidenced by peribronchial air. Although this is not

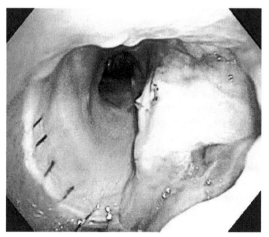

Fig. 6. Severe necrosis and dehiscence. Note the separation of graft from native airway with tissue loss along the posterior wall.

uncommon immediately after a transplant, additional factors may alert one to a dehiscence. Extensive amounts of peribronchial air in conjunction with bronchial wall abnormalities, dissection into the mediastinum, or fascial planes should increase a clinician's concern.[85–87]

The gold standard for diagnosis is bronchoscopy, because radiographic studies cannot reliably image the mucosa. In the setting of severe necrosis, it may be difficult to see the actual site of dehiscence; however, there are several clues seen endoscopically. Significant necrosis and loose sutures can be evidence that the anastomosis is at risk, presently dehiscing, or has already dehisced. Ultimately, the management of dehiscence will vary based on its severity. The most severe cases may require an open surgical repair, flap bronchoplasty, or even retransplantation, although this is quite risky, with less than ideal results.[22]

No intervention except close observation is typically required for grade I and II bronchial dehiscence, although antibiotic regimens, including inhaled delivery methods, may be practical.

Fortunately, grade III and IV bronchial dehiscence are not common, approximately 1.6% in the authors' experience, because they can have devastating complications. Most patients with grade III or IV dehiscence eventually develop infection, and this is the usual source of mortality. The severity of the dehiscence and its clinical impact will dictate the management. Both bronchoscopic and surgical techniques exist for the treatment, although more invasive approaches are fraught with a high morbidity and mortality. Surgical options for repair include reanastomosis, a flap bronchoplasty, or in severe cases, a retransplantation.[22]

Bronchoscopic techniques described include cyanoacrylate glue, growth factors, and autologous platelet-derived factors. Although some reports have been successful, the general impression in these techniques is lacking.[88]

Using the temporary placement of noncovered SEMS, the authors' institution has described a novel bronchoscopic approach for grade III and IV dehiscence (**Fig. 7**). This technique uses the propensity to cause granulation tissue, a well-known complication of SEMS, as an advantage. Once airway patency is optimized with gently dilation and/or debulking, a noncovered SEMS is deployed in the airway, covering the dehiscence, and closely followed. Healing may be appreciated in as little as 1 week with a removal/replacement occurring once epithelialization/granulation tissue develops, typically within a few weeks. Several cycles of this technique have demonstrated healing of the bronchial wall. In the authors' experience, 37.5 days was the mean time to removal.[82]

Incumbent in this technique is expertise not only in placing but also (and possibly more importantly)

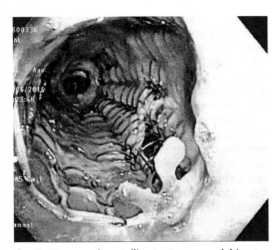

Fig. 7. Uncovered metallic stent over a dehiscence with a mediastinal fistula noted in the medial wall of the right main bronchus (see **Fig. 6**).

in removal of the SEMS. Improper stent placement or manipulation can easily extend the airway injury as can an overaggressive removal, so great care must be taken. Complications such as stenosis and malacia are more frequently encountered even if the dehiscence is successfully closed. Continued close surveillance is recommended.

EXOPHYTIC GRANULATION TISSUE

In about 7% to 24% of lung-transplant patients, benign hyperplastic endoluminal granulation tissue may cause significant airway obstruction[89] and typically occurs at the anastomotic site a few months after transplantation.[57]

The cause of the formation of the hyperplastic tissue may be related to ischemia and inflammation with a subsequent remodeling process.[57,90] Similar to keloid reactions, an exaggerated immune response may be present. Anastomotic infections, especially *Aspergillus*, may intensify its formation.[21] Also, therapeutic interventions, such as airway stenting, promote the formation of granulation tissue.[82,90] After stent placement, the estimated incidence of granulation tissue formation is around 12% to 36%.[66,91] The incidence of granulation tissue formation related to airway stents has been described to be less in posttransplant patients, theoretically related to the immunosuppressant medications used.[92]

Depending on the degree of airway obstruction, excessive granulation tissue formation may present with progressive dyspnea, cough, hypoxia, hemoptysis, decreased secretions clearance, or postobstructive pneumonia.[1,57] Decreasing spirometry values may be seen. Chest CT may show the obstructive granulation tissue at the bronchi that is typically confirmed by direct visualization of the airway.

Its management requires a multidisciplinary approach, and often multiple procedures are needed because of its tendency to recur. Debridement is the management of choice. Based on the amount of granulation tissue, the degree of obstruction, and the location, several techniques for debridement may be used, including forceps (flexible or rigid), cryotherapy, APC, electrocautery, or laser.[1,37,91,93,94]

Cryotherapy, APC, and laser techniques have been described elsewhere and are beyond the scope of this article. Cryotherapy advantages are the safety profile, the cryosensitivity of granulation tissue, its excellent hemostasis, and the ability of using high-oxygen concentrations. Cryotherapy causes cell lysis due to cellular crystallization. Although historically its use is described as a delayed effect, cryoablation of endobronchial tissue with cryo-recanalization can result in an immediate therapy.[95,96] Furthermore, cryotherapy may be used around granulation tissue in silicone stents without the risk of ignition. APC, electrocautery, and Nd:YAG laser have also been described successfully for granulation tissue management after lung transplantation.

Despite the above methods, recurrence is common and difficult to treat. Retrospectives studies have shown the use of high-dose-rate endobronchial brachytherapy (HDR-EB) for recalcitrant cases. By using Iridium-192, a high dose of conformal dose of ionizing radiation is used to treat excessive granulation tissue at the anastomosis and related to endobronchial stents, while minimizing radiation exposure to the surrounding structures.[57,90] Serious and fatal complications, such as massive hemoptysis, have been described with HDR-EB, and extreme caution must be used when considering this approach.[76]

Approaches to prevent the formation of granulation tissue have been used. Specifically, topical mitomycin-C may be applied to reduce the proliferation of granulation tissue due to its ability to inhibit the proliferation of fibroblast.[97,98] The antineoplastic agent is applied at the airway after granulation tissue debridement by any of the above-mentioned methods to reduce its recurrence.[98,99] A dose from 0.5 to 1 mg/mL may be used via pledget and swabbed to the area for few minutes.[76] Randomized trials are lacking; however, given the safety profile of mitomycin-C and its potential advantages, mitomycin-C is frequently used.

TRACHEOBRONCHOMALACIA

Tracheomalacia and bronchomalacia have been defined as a luminal narrowing of 50% or more on expiration.[61] The diameter reduction may be related to the loss of cartilaginous support or because of excessive dynamic airway collapse. It may be seen diffusely after lung transplantation, at the anastomotic site, or associated with bronchial stenosis. Pathologic airway cartilage changes have been described, but its pathophysiology is poorly understood. The cartilage may be damaged by peritransplant ischemia or infections.

Signs and symptoms include cough, dyspnea, recurrent infections, wheezing, and the inability to clear secretions. A common "barking" cough has been described. Reductions in the FEV1, forced expiratory flow at 25% to 75%, and a low peak expiratory flow rate may be encountered. The flow-volume loops may show a variable obstruction, more marked during expiration. Bronchoscopic airway examination is the gold standard

for diagnosis; however, a dynamic CT of the chest may suggest the process.[51,61,74]

Tracheobronchomalacia management is a therapeutic dilemma. The intervention will depend on the severity of its presentation. Most of the recommendations are extrapolated from non-transplant-related malacia. Medical management includes pulmonary hygiene, mucolytics, and noninvasive positive pressure ventilation.[1,100] In cases with severe functional impairment and symptoms despite medical interventions, airway stenting may be used. The stent will allow restoring and maintaining airway patency, improving secretions clearance, and improving infection. Small studies have shown that stent placement for transplant-related bronchomalacia improves spirometry values.[56] Silicone stents are preferred, and once deployed, close surveillance is needed. Rarely, after all other alternatives have been exhausted, an SEMS may be used, taking into consideration the concerns about metallic stents and benign diseases.[76]

FISTULAS

Airway fistulas after lung transplantation are uncommon, but a very challenging complication to treat. Fistulas between the airway and the pleura, mediastinum, aorta, pulmonary arteries, and the left atrium have been described.[1,96,101–105] Fortunately, given the devastating complications, fistulas are quite rare.

A bronchopleural fistula is rarely seen, is probably related to bronchial ischemia, is associated with high morbidity and mortality, and typically occurs early in the postoperative period. A bronchopleural fistula may present as dyspnea, hypotension, sepsis, pneumothorax including tension, subcutaneous emphysema, or persistent air leaks. It is usually encountered in the setting of dehiscence. Main points on its management are infection control with antibiotics and thoracostomy drainage. Endoscopic closure of the fistula may be attempted, as the initial choice, and usually the success depends on the size and location. Endoscopic techniques include cyanoacrylate glue, fibrinogen plus thrombin, or bronchial stents. Also, intrabronchial one-way valves may be an option. Surgical options include flaps, open drainage, or thoracoplasty.[1,76,100]

A bronchomediastinal fistula with or without dehiscence has a high mortality due to sepsis.[2] The presentation may be as bacteremia, sepsis, mediastinitis, mediastinal abscess, or cavitation. They are more commonly seen at the anastomosis site but may occur at any place in the airway (see **Fig. 7**).

Bronchovascular fistulas are very rare and are associated with high mortality. A minor premonitory hemoptysis episode may be seen, followed by a fatal bleed. A fistula should be suspected in cases of infectious complications (*Aspergillus*) combined with moderate hemoptysis.[1,76,106] In addition to hemoptysis, air embolism and sepsis have been described.[100,107] Its management literature is limited to case reports of pneumonectomy and bilobectomy.

ANASTOMOTIC INFECTIONS

In lung transplantation, the susceptibility to infections is determined by various factors, including the degree of immunosuppression, use of steroids, airway anatomy, ischemic complications, suture misfortunes, impaired mucociliary function, altered phagocytosis in alveolar macrophages, interrupted lymphatic drainage, direct communication of the lungs with the atmosphere, and the lack of tracheobronchial cough reflex due to organ denervation.[108,109] Furthermore, the allograft is exposed not only to the external environment but also to the flora of the native and donor's airways.[110] Also, many patients even in the pretransplant period are already colonized with multi-drug-resistant organisms.

Overall, infections are common after lung transplantation. An incidence of 34% to 59% has been described and is significantly higher when compared with other solid organ transplants.[111] Bacterial and fungal infections are most frequently seen in the first month after transplant, while viral infections are more common in the second and third postoperative months.[111]

Bacterial pneumonia is the most common infection in lung transplant recipients. About 75% of lung-transplant patients will develop a bacterial pneumonia within 3 months after transplantation.[109]

Endobronchial infections are common as well, and usually opportunistic infections are involved. The infection may involve the entire airway, such as bronchitis or tracheitis, or the anastomosis area. *Pseudomonas* and *Staphylococcus* are the most frequent acquired bacterial infections.[1,112] Saprophytic fungal organisms are also quite common. *Aspergillus* is the most frequently involved. Other reported fungal organisms include *Cladosporium*, *Candida*, *Zygomycetes* (mucormycosis), and *Scedosporium* species.

Aspergillus colonizes about 20% of lung-transplant patients in the immediate postoperative period. Clinically, *Aspergillus* infection posttransplant may present as invasive pulmonary aspergillosis, colonization, or tracheobronchitis, and precise diagnosis of these syndromes can be very difficult.[113] Locally invasive or disseminated *Aspergillus* infection accounts for 2% to 33% of infections following lung transplantation and has a high reported mortality. Airway colonization with *Aspergillus fumigatus* in the first 6 months posttransplant has a 11-fold increased risk of developing invasive disease.[109] *Aspergillus* also is associated with an ulcerative tracheobronchitis that can lead to anastomotic dehiscence.[109] Anastomotic complications are more common in patients with *Aspergillus* infection.[113,114]

Anastomotic infections represent an airway complication and may predispose to all the other AC as well. The mechanisms are not well understood, but infection may lead to dehiscence, fistula formation, stenosis, or granulation tissue formation, and if it invades the bronchial wall directly, airway collapse and malacia.

Diagnosis of anastomotic infections is usually done at bronchoscopy. The infections tend to be relatively asymptomatic, although some patients may complain of fever, cough, secretions, wheezing, and/or hemoptysis. At bronchoscopic examination, airway erythema, ulceration, and pseudomembranes may be seen. Positive cultures are vital to identifying the organism and tailor treatment, especially in fungal causes.

Treatment includes bronchoscopic debridement of devitalized tissue and antibiotic therapy. With regards to fungal infections, given the potential consequences of *Aspergillus* colonization or infection, prevention is key. In the first 6 months after transplant, most programs routinely use antifungal prophylaxis. Voriconazole, itraconazole, and inhaled amphotericin-B formulas are the most commonly used chemotherapy agents.[113,114]

MANAGEMENT SUMMARY

Management of AC is complicated. Many modalities are available and which modality is optimal may not be clear, because no randomized trials exist to direct the clinician. The optimal management is a multidisciplinary approach performed by individuals experienced in not only the techniques discussed but also the nuances of a posttransplant patient.

BRONCHIAL ARTERY REVASCULARIZATION

As previously discussed, routine lung transplantation does not restore the bronchial artery supply, posing a unique problem in this population. An attempt to improve this process was developed and studied. Allowing the anastomosis of bronchial arteries and preservation of blood flow

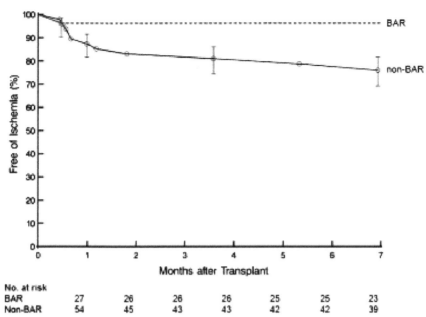

Fig. 8. Bronchial artery revascularization associated with less ischemia. (*From* Pettersson GB, Karam K, Thuita L, et al. Comparative study of bronchial artery revascularization in lung transplantation. J Thorac Cardiovasc Surg 2013;146(4):894–900.e3; with permission.)

to the airways showed early promising results. BAR has been described as a successful alternative in small series.[115–118] In the largest series of BAR to date, a single institution demonstrated improved survival over sequential bilateral lung transplantation.[119,120]

The BAR procedure has been described in detail in the referenced articles; however, a brief summary has merit in this review. During BAR, the donor lungs are procured en bloc via sternotomy, including both the esophagus and the descending aorta, thus securing inclusion of the retroesophageal right

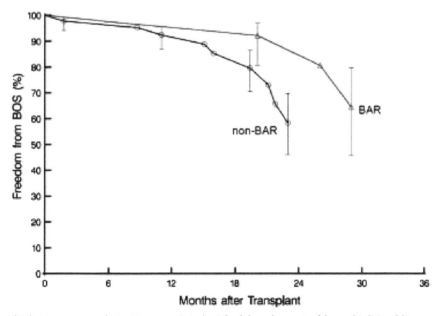

Fig. 9. Bronchial artery revascularization associated with delayed onset of bronchiolitis obliterans syndrome. (*From* Pettersson GB, Karam K, Thuita L, et al. Comparative study of bronchial artery revascularization in lung transplantation. J Thorac Cardiovasc Surg 2013;146(4):894–900.e3; with permission.)

intercostobronchial artery. One internal thoracic artery is harvested. When double-lung transplantation is performed, cardiopulmonary bypass (CPB) is used with a tracheal anastomosis. For the en bloc transplants, BAR anastomoses are performed first, followed by the trachea, pulmonary trunk, and left atrium. The internal thoracic artery is then anastomosed to at least 1 bronchial artery ostia in the donor descending aorta. Single-lung transplantation is not performed on CPB and the bronchial anastomosis occurs at the secondary carina, as in non-BAR transplants, and is the final anastomosis after giving 10,000 IU of heparin and pulmonary artery reperfusion.[115,116,121–126]

This technique was recently readdressed at the authors' institution. The actual reanastomosis was successful in 26 of 27 patients. This pilot showed that this technique was feasible, associated with less airway ischemia, and required no airway interventions (**Fig. 8**). A higher risk of bleeding was found, but safety was comparable between BAR and non-BAR patients. Additional findings that may show future relevance included less early rejection, fewer infections, and delay of BOS (**Fig. 9**). Although these findings are encouraging, a multicenter study is needed to firmly establish these benefits.[127]

SUMMARY

Lung transplant anatomy and the techniques associated with it pose a unique problem in transplantation. Many causes may be responsible for causing AC and similarly many techniques are available to deal with these. AC can have a significant impact on the quality of life of the patient after transplantation. Frequent visits to specialists, interventions, and recurrence of symptoms can be quite frustrating, and although bronchoscopic interventions may significantly improve the patient's symptoms and FEV1, these repeated visits and procedures could be troubling, time-consuming, and costly. Many patients who undergo a transplant do so understanding that their survival may not be significantly extended, but rather they will have an improved quality of life. The symptoms associated with AC as well as the need for frequent procedures no doubt have a detrimental effect on this proposed benefit. The impact on survival may not be as apparent. The overall survival after a lung transplant is approximately 50% at 5 years. Patients with treated anastomotic AC have equivalent early rates of mortality as those patients without complications. There does appear to be an increased late risk beginning at approximately 18 months. In patients who received no treatment for their AC, there was a

higher early mortality but their late risk was equivalent to patients who had no AC. Lung-transplant patients are varied and complex and so are their complications; this is particularly true relating to AC. Multiple presentations of AC are described and as such a myriad of management strategies may be used. Different techniques are used due to the differences in the types of complications, but many yield a successful outcome. Improvements in many areas, such as surgical techniques, peri-procedural and intensive care unit management, immunosuppression, endoscopic treatments, and donor and recipient selection, are likely to lead to optimal outcomes. Currently, there are no blinded, randomized control trials demonstrating a superior algorithm of management of AC. The management of each individual complication requires an individualized multidisciplinary approach by a team with considerable expertise and experience. It is hoped that future studies in this heterogeneous population will lead to optimal treatment in this complex patient group.

REFERENCES

1. Santacruz JF, Mehta AC. Airway complications and management after lung transplantation: ischemia, dehiscence, and stenosis. Proc Am Thorac Soc 2009;6(1):79–93.
2. Shennib H, Massard G. Airway complications in lung transplantation. Ann Thorac Surg 1994;57(2): 506–11.
3. Hasegawa T, Iacono AT, Orons PD, et al. Segmental nonanastomotic bronchial stenosis after lung transplantation. Ann Thorac Surg 2000;69(4): 1020–4.
4. Schmid RA, Boehler A, Speich R, et al. Bronchial anastomotic complications following lung transplantation: still a major cause of morbidity? Eur Respir J 1997;10(12):2872–5.
5. Wildevuur CR, Benfield JR. A review of 23 human lung transplantations by 20 surgeons. Ann Thorac Surg 1970;9(6):489–515.
6. Kapoor BS, May B, Panu N, et al. Endobronchial stent placement for the management of airway complications after lung transplantation. J Vasc Interv Radiol 2007;18(5):629–32.
7. Shah SS, Karnak D, Minai O, et al. Symptomatic narrowing or atresia of bronchus intermedius following lung transplantation vanishing bronchus intermedius syndrome (VBIS). Chest J 2006; 130(4_MeetingAbstracts):236S. a-236S. Available at: http://journal.publications.chestnet.org/article.aspx?articleID=1215386.
8. Samano MN, Minamoto H, Junqueira JJ, et al. Bronchial complications following lung transplantation. Transplant Proc 2009;41(3):921–6.

9. Van De Wauwer C, Van Raemdonck D, Verleden GM, et al. Risk factors for airway complications within the first year after lung transplantation. Eur J Cardiothorac Surg 2007;31(4):703–10.

10. Murthy SC, Blackstone EH, Gildea TR, et al. Impact of anastomotic airway complications after lung transplantation. Ann Thorac Surg 2007;84(2):401–9, 409. e1–4.

11. Shofer SL, Wahidi MM, Davis WA, et al. Significance of and risk factors for the development of central airway stenosis after lung transplantation. Am J Transplant 2013;13(2):383–9.

12. Dutau H, Vandemoortele T, Laroumagne S, et al. A new endoscopic standardized grading system for macroscopic central airway complications following lung transplantation: the MDS classification. Eur J Cardiothorac Surg 2014;45(2):e33–8.

13. Herrera JM, McNeil KD, Higgins RS, et al. Airway complications after lung transplantation: treatment and long-term outcome. Ann Thorac Surg 2001; 71(3):989–93 [discussion: 993–4].

14. Meyers BF, de la Morena M, Sweet SC, et al. Primary graft dysfunction and other selected complications of lung transplantation: a single-center experience of 983 patients. J Thorac Cardiovasc Surg 2005;129(6):1421–9.

15. Garfein ES, McGregor CC, Galantowicz ME, et al. Deleterious effects of telescoped bronchial anastomosis in single and bilateral lung transplantation. Ann Transplant 2000;5(1):5–11.

16. Schroder C, Scholl F, Daon E, et al. A modified bronchial anastomosis technique for lung transplantation. Ann Thorac Surg 2003;75(6):1697–704.

17. Alvarez A, Algar J, Santos F, et al. Airway complications after lung transplantation: a review of 151 anastomoses. Eur J Cardiothorac Surg 2001;19(4): 381–7.

18. Mason DP, Brown CR, Murthy SC, et al. Growing single-center experience with lung transplantation using donation after cardiac death. Ann Thorac Surg 2012;94(2):406–11 [discussion: 411–2].

19. De Oliveira NC, Osaki S, Maloney JD, et al. Lung transplantation with donation after cardiac death donors: long-term follow-up in a single center. J Thorac Cardiovasc Surg 2010;139(5):1306–15.

20. Ruttmann E, Ulmer H, Marchese M, et al. Evaluation of factors damaging the bronchial wall in lung transplantation. J Heart Lung Transplant 2005;24(3):275–81.

21. Mulligan MS. Endoscopic management of airway complications after lung transplantation. Chest Surg Clin N Am 2001;11(4):907–15.

22. Kshettry VR, Kroshus TJ, Hertz MI, et al. Early and late airway complications after lung transplantation: Incidence and management. Ann Thorac Surg 1997;63(6):1576–83.

23. Murthy SC, Gildea TR, Machuzak MS. Anastomotic airway complications after lung transplantation. Curr Opin Organ Transplant 2010;15(5):582–7.

24. Schafers HJ, Wagner TO, Demertzis S, et al. Preoperative corticosteroids. A contraindication to lung transplantation? Chest 1992;102(5):1522–5.

25. Colquhoun IW, Gascoigne AD, Au J, et al. Airway complications after pulmonary transplantation. Ann Thorac Surg 1994;57(1):141–5.

26. Schafers HJ, Haverich A, Wagner TO, et al. Decreased incidence of bronchial complications following lung transplantation. Eur J Cardiothorac Surg 1992;6(4):174–8 [discussion: 179].

27. Groetzner J, Kur F, Spelsberg F, et al. Airway anastomosis complications in de novo lung transplantation with sirolimus-based immunosuppression. J Heart Lung Transplant 2004;23(5):632–8.

28. Date H, Trulock EP, Arcidi JM, et al. Improved airway healing after lung transplantation. an analysis of 348 bronchial anastomoses. J Thorac Cardiovasc Surg 1995;110(5):1424–32 [discussion: 1432–3].

29. Khaghani A, Tadjkarimi S, al-Kattan K, et al. Wrapping the anastomosis with omentum or an internal mammary artery pedicle does not improve bronchial healing after single lung transplantation: results of a randomized clinical trial. J Heart Lung Transplant 1994;13(5):767–73.

30. Griffith BP, Magee MJ, Gonzalez IF, et al. Anastomotic pitfalls in lung transplantation. J Thorac Cardiovasc Surg 1994;107(3):743–53 [discussion: 753–4].

31. Garfein ES, Ginsberg ME, Gorenstein L, et al. Superiority of end-to-end versus telescoped bronchial anastomosis in single lung transplantation for pulmonary emphysema. J Thorac Cardiovasc Surg 2001;121(1):149–54.

32. Choong CK, Sweet SC, Zoole JB, et al. Bronchial airway anastomotic complications after pediatric lung transplantation: incidence, cause, management, and outcome. J Thorac Cardiovasc Surg 2006;131(1):198–203.

33. Davis RD Jr, Pasque MK. Pulmonary transplantation. Ann Surg 1995;221(1):14–28.

34. de Pablo A, Lopez S, Ussetti P, et al. Lung transplant therapy for suppurative diseases. Arch Bronconeumol 2005;41(5):255–9.

35. Bloom RD, Goldberg LR, Wang AY, et al. An overview of solid organ transplantation. Clin Chest Med 2005;26(4):529–43, v.

36. Park SJ, Nguyen DQ, Savik K, et al. Pre-transplant corticosteroid use and outcome in lung transplantation. J Heart Lung Transplant 2001;20(3):304–9.

37. Kaditis AG, Gondor M, Nixon PA, et al. Airway complications following pediatric lung and heart-lung transplantation. Am J Respir Crit Care Med 2000; 162(1):301–9.

38. McAnally KJ, Valentine VG, LaPlace SG, et al. Effect of pre-transplantation prednisone on survival after lung transplantation. J Heart Lung Transplant 2006;25(1):67–74.

39. King-Biggs MB, Dunitz JM, Park SJ, et al. Airway anastomotic dehiscence associated with use of sirolimus immediately after lung transplantation. Transplantation 2003;75(9):1437–43.

40. Yokomise H, Cardoso PF, Kato H, et al. The effect of pulmonary arterial flow and positive end-expiratory pressure on retrograde bronchial mucosal blood flow. J Thorac Cardiovasc Surg 1991;101(2):201–8.

41. Porhownik NR. Airway complications post lung transplantation. Curr Opin Pulm Med 2013;19(2): 174–80.

42. Eberlein M, Arnaoutakis GJ, Yarmus L, et al. The effect of lung size mismatch on complications and resource utilization after bilateral lung transplantation. J Heart Lung Transplant 2012;31(5):492–500.

43. Lonchyna VA, Arcidi JM Jr, Garrity ER Jr, et al. Refractory post-transplant airway strictures: successful management with wire stents. Eur J Cardiothorac Surg 1999;15(6):842–9 [discussion: 849–50].

44. Christie JD, Carby M, Bag R, et al. Report of the ISHLT working group on primary lung graft dysfunction part II: definition. A consensus statement of the international society for heart and lung transplantation. J Heart Lung Transplant 2005;24(10):1454–9.

45. Couraud L, Nashef SA, Nicolini P, et al. Classification of airway anastomotic healing. Eur J Cardiothorac Surg 1992;6(9):496–7.

46. Thistlethwaite PA, Yung G, Kemp A, et al. Airway stenoses after lung transplantation: incidence, management, and outcome. J Thorac Cardiovasc Surg 2008;136(6):1569–75.

47. De Gracia J, Culebras M, Alvarez A, et al. Bronchoscopic balloon dilatation in the management of bronchial stenosis following lung transplantation. Respir Med 2007;101(1):27–33.

48. Marulli G, Loy M, Rizzardi G, et al. Surgical treatment of posttransplant bronchial stenoses: case reports. Transplant Proc 2007;39(6):1973–5.

49. Castleberry AW, Worni M, Kuchibhatla M, et al. A comparative analysis of bronchial stricture after lung transplantation in recipients with and without early acute rejection. Ann Thorac Surg 2013; 96(3):1008–17 [discussion: 1017–8].

50. Souilamas R, Wermert D, Guillemain R, et al. Uncommon combined treatment of nonanastomotic bronchial stenosis after lung transplantation. J Bronchology Interv Pulmonol 2008;15(1):54–5. http://dx.doi.org/10.1097/LBR.0b013e318162c415.

51. Krishnam MS, Suh RD, Tomasian A, et al. Postoperative complications of lung transplantation: radiologic findings along a time continuum. Radiographics 2007;27(4):957–74.

52. Neagos GR, Martinez FJ, Deeb GM, et al. Diagnosis of unilateral mainstem bronchial obstruction following single-lung transplantation with routine spirometry. Chest 1993;103(4):1255–8.

53. Anzueto A, Levine SM, Tillis WP, et al. Use of the flow-volume loop in the diagnosis of bronchial stenosis after single lung transplantation. Chest 1994; 105(3):934–6.

54. Garg K, Zamora MR, Tuder R, et al. Lung transplantation: indications, donor and recipient selection, and imaging of complications. Radiographics 1996;16(2):355–67.

55. Quint LE, Whyte RI, Kazerooni EA, et al. Stenosis of the central airways: evaluation by using helical CT with multiplanar reconstructions. Radiology 1995; 194(3):871–7.

56. Chhajed PN, Malouf MA, Tamm M, et al. Interventional bronchoscopy for the management of airway complications following lung transplantation. Chest 2001;120(6):1894–9.

57. Tendulkar RD, Fleming PA, Reddy CA, et al. High-dose-rate endobronchial brachytherapy for recurrent airway obstruction from hyperplastic granulation tissue. Int J Radiat Oncol Biol Phys 2008;70(3):701–6.

58. Mayse ML, Greenheck J, Friedman M, et al. Successful bronchoscopic balloon dilation of nonmalignant tracheobronchial obstruction without fluoroscopy. Chest 2004;126(2):634–7.

59. Mathur PN, Wolf KM, Busk MF, et al. Fiberoptic bronchoscopic cryotherapy in the management of tracheobronchial obstruction. Chest 1996;110(3): 718–23.

60. McArdle JR, Gildea TR, Mehta AC. Balloon bronchoplasty: its indications, benefits, and complications. J Bronchology Interv Pulmonol 2005;12(2): 123–7. http://dx.doi.org/10.1097/01.laboratory. 0000159783.34078.3d.

61. Simoff M, Sterman D, Ernst A, editors. Thoracic endoscopy. Advances in interventional pulmonology. Malden (MA): Blackwell Publishing; 2006.

62. Dutau H, Vandemoortele T, Breen DP. Rigid bronchoscopy. Clin Chest Med 2013;34(3):427–35.

63. Tremblay A, Coulter TD, Mehta AC. Modification of a mucosal-sparing technique using electrocautery and balloon dilatation in the endoscopic management of web-like benign airway stenosis. J Bronchology Interv Pulmonol 2003;10(4): 268–71.

64. Verhaeghe W, Noppen M, Meysman M, et al. Rapid healing of endobronchial tuberculosis by local endoscopic injection of corticosteroids. Monaldi Arch Chest Dis 1996;51(5):391–3.

65. Cosano-Povedano J, Muñoz-Cabrera L, Jurado-Gámez B, et al. Topical mitomycin C for recurrent bronchial stenosis after lung transplantation: a report of 2 cases. J Bronchology Interv Pulmonol 2008;15(4):281–3. http://dx.doi.org/10.1097/LBR.0b013e3181879e3a.

66. Saad CP, Ghamande SA, Minai OA, et al. The role of self-expandable metallic stents for the treatment of airway complications after lung transplantation. Transplantation 2003;75(9):1532–8.

67. Bolliger CT, Sutedja TG, Strausz J, et al. Therapeutic bronchoscopy with immediate effect: laser, electrocautery, argon plasma coagulation and stents. Eur Respir J 2006;27(6):1258–71.

68. Grosu HB, Eapen GA, Morice RC, et al. Stents are associated with increased risk of respiratory infections in patients undergoing airway interventions for malignant airways disease. Chest 2013;144(2):441–9.

69. Doyle DJ, Abdelmalak B, Machuzak M, et al. Anesthesia and airway management for removing pulmonary self-expanding metallic stents. J Clin Anesth 2009;21(7):529–32.

70. Murthy SC, Gildea TR, Mehta AC. Removal of self-expandable metallic stents: is it possible? Semin Respir Crit Care Med 2004;25(4):381–5.

71. Lunn W, Feller-Kopman D, Wahidi M, et al. Endoscopic removal of metallic airway stents. Chest 2005;127(6):2106–12.

72. Fernandez-Bussy S, Akindipe O, Kulkarni V, et al. Clinical experience with a new removable tracheobronchial stent in the management of airway complications after lung transplantation. J Heart Lung Transplant 2009;28(7):683–8.

73. Madden BP, Loke TK, Sheth AC. Do expandable metallic airway stents have a role in the management of patients with benign tracheobronchial disease? Ann Thorac Surg 2006;82(1):274–8.

74. Murgu SD, Colt HG. Complications of silicone stent insertion in patients with expiratory central airway collapse. Ann Thorac Surg 2007;84(6):1870–7.

75. Gildea TR, Murthy SC, Sahoo D, et al. Performance of a self-expanding silicone stent in palliation of benign airway conditions. Chest 2006;130(5):1419–23.

76. Machuzak M. Management of posttransplant disorders. In: Ernst A, Herth FJ, editors. Principles and practice of interventional pulmonology. New York: Springer Science+Business Media; 2013. p. 463.

77. Alraiyes AH, Machuzak MS, Gildea TR. Intussusception technique of intrabronchial silicone stents: description of technique and a case report. J Bronchology Interv Pulmonol 2013;20(4):342–4.

78. Lari SM, Gonin F, Colchen A. The management of bronchus intermedius complications after lung transplantation: a retrospective study. J Cardiothorac Surg 2012;7:8. http://dx.doi.org/10.1186/1749-8090-7-8.

79. Sundset A, Lund MB, Hansen G, et al. Airway complications after lung transplantation: long-term outcome of silicone stenting. Respiration 2012;83(3):245–8.

80. Wang K, Mehta A, Turner J, editors. Flexible bronchoscopy. 2nd edition. Malden (MA): Blackwell Publishing; 2004.

81. Dutau H, Cavailles A, Sakr L, et al. A retrospective study of silicone stent placement for management of anastomotic airway complications in lung transplant recipients: short- and long-term outcomes. J Heart Lung Transplant 2010;29(6):658–64.

82. Mughal MM, Gildea TR, Murthy S, et al. Short-term deployment of self-expanding metallic stents facilitates healing of bronchial dehiscence. Am J Respir Crit Care Med 2005;172(6):768–71.

83. Usuda K, Gildea TR, Pandya C, et al. Bronchial dehiscence. J Bronchology Interv Pulmonol 2005;12(3):164–5. http://dx.doi.org/10.1097/01.lab.0000158968.46655.e3.

84. Herman SJ, Weisbrod GL, Weisbrod L, et al. Chest radiographic findings after bilateral lung transplantation. AJR Am J Roentgenol 1989;153(6):1181–5.

85. Semenkovich JW, Glazer HS, Anderson DC, et al. Bronchial dehiscence in lung transplantation: CT evaluation. Radiology 1995;194(1):205–8.

86. O'Donovan PB. Imaging of complications of lung transplantation. Radiographics 1993;13(4):787–96.

87. Schlueter FJ, Semenkovich JW, Glazer HS, et al. Bronchial dehiscence after lung transplantation: correlation of CT findings with clinical outcome. Radiology 1996;199(3):849–54.

88. Maloney JD, Weigel TL, Love RB. Endoscopic repair of bronchial dehiscence after lung transplantation. Ann Thorac Surg 2001;72(6):2109–11.

89. Meyer A, Warszawski-Baumann A, Baumann R, et al. HDR brachytherapy: an option for preventing nonmalignant obstruction in patients after lung transplantation. Strahlenther Onkol 2012;188(12):1085–90.

90. Kennedy AS, Sonett JR, Orens JB, et al. High dose rate brachytherapy to prevent recurrent benign hyperplasia in lung transplant bronchi: theoretical and clinical considerations. J Heart Lung Transplant 2000;19(2):155–9.

91. Madden BP, Kumar P, Sayer R, et al. Successful resection of obstructing airway granulation tissue following lung transplantation using endobronchial laser (Nd:YAG) therapy. Eur J Cardiothorac Surg 1997;12(3):480–5.

92. Redmond J, Diamond J, Dunn J, et al. Rigid bronchoscopic management of complications related to endobronchial stents after lung transplantation. Ann Otol Rhinol Laryngol 2013;122(3):183–9.

93. Maiwand MO, Zehr KJ, Dyke CM, et al. The role of cryotherapy for airway complications after lung and heart-lung transplantation. Eur J Cardiothorac Surg 1997;12(4):549–54.

94. Keller CA, Hinerman R, Singh A, et al. The use of endoscopic argon plasma coagulation in airway complications after solid organ transplantation. Chest 2001;119(6):1968–75.

95. Yilmaz A, Aktas Z, Alici IO, et al. Cryorecanalization: keys to success. Surg Endosc 2012;26(10): 2969–74.

96. Guth S, Mayer E, Fischer B, et al. Bilobectomy for massive hemoptysis after bilateral lung transplantation. J Thorac Cardiovasc Surg 2001;121(6):1194–5.

97. Ubell ML, Ettema SL, Toohill RJ, et al. Mitomycin-c application in airway stenosis surgery: analysis of safety and costs. Otolaryngol Head Neck Surg 2006;134(3):403–6.

98. Erard AC, Monnier P, Spiliopoulos A, et al. Mitomycin C for control of recurrent bronchial stenosis: a case report. Chest 2001;120(6):2103–5.

99. Penafiel A, Lee P, Hsu A, et al. Topical mitomycin-C for obstructing endobronchial granuloma. Ann Thorac Surg 2006;82(3):e22–3.

100. Puchalski J, Lee HJ, Sterman DH. Airway complications following lung transplantation. Clin Chest Med 2011;32(2):357–66.

101. Chang CC, Hsu HH, Kuo SW, et al. Bronchoscopic gluing for post-lung-transplant bronchopleural fistula. Eur J Cardiothorac Surg 2007;31(2):328–30.

102. Mora G, de Pablo A, Garcia-Gallo CL, et al. Is endoscopic treatment of bronchopleural fistula useful? Arch Bronconeumol 2006;42(8):394–8.

103. Hoff SJ, Johnson JE, Frist WH. Aortobronchial fistula after unilateral lung transplantation. Ann Thorac Surg 1993;56(6):1402–3.

104. Karmy-Jones R, Vallieres E, Culver B, et al. Bronchial-atrial fistula after lung transplant resulting in fatal air embolism. Ann Thorac Surg 1999;67(2): 550–1.

105. Rea F, Marulli G, Loy M, et al. Salvage right pneumonectomy in a patient with bronchial-pulmonary artery fistula after bilateral sequential lung transplantation. J Heart Lung Transplant 2006;25(11): 1383–6.

106. Verleden GM, Vos R, van Raemdonck D, et al. Pulmonary infection defense after lung transplantation: does airway ischemia play a role? Curr Opin Organ Transplant 2010;15(5):568–71.

107. Knight J, Elwing JM, Milstone A. Bronchovascular fistula formation: a rare airway complication after lung transplantation. J Heart Lung Transplant 2008;27(10):1179–85.

108. Parada MT, Alba A, Sepulveda C. Early and late infections in lung transplantation patients. Transplant Proc 2010;42(1):333–5.

109. Ahuja J, Kanne JP. Thoracic infections in immunocompromised patients. Radiol Clin North Am 2014;52(1):121–36.

110. Nunley DR, Gal AA, Vega JD, et al. Saprophytic fungal infections and complications involving the bronchial anastomosis following human lung transplantation. Chest 2002;122(4):1185–91.

111. Diez Martinez P, Pakkal M, Prenovault J, et al. Postoperative imaging after lung transplantation. Clin Imaging 2013;37(4):617–23.

112. Shteinberg M, Raviv Y, Bishara J, et al. The impact of fluoroquinolone resistance of gram-negative bacteria in respiratory secretions on the outcome of lung transplant (non-cystic fibrosis) recipients. Clin Transplant 2012;26(6):884–90.

113. Felton TW, Roberts SA, Isalska B, et al. Isolation of aspergillus species from the airway of lung transplant recipients is associated with excess mortality. J Infect 2012;65(4):350–6.

114. Weder W, Inci I, Korom S, et al. Airway complications after lung transplantation: Risk factors, prevention and outcome. Eur J Cardiothorac Surg 2009;35(2):293–8 [discussion: 298].

115. Couraud L, Baudet E, Martigne C, et al. Bronchial revascularization in double-lung transplantation: a series of 8 patients. Bordeaux Lung and Heart-Lung Transplant Group. Ann Thorac Surg 1992; 53(1):88–94.

116. Couraud L, Baudet E, Nashef SA, et al. Lung transplantation with bronchial revascularisation. Surgical anatomy, operative technique and early results. Eur J Cardiothorac Surg 1992;6(9):490–5.

117. Daly RC, McGregor CG. Routine immediate direct bronchial artery revascularization for single-lung transplantation. Ann Thorac Surg 1994;57(6): 1446–52.

118. Pettersson G, Arendrup H, Mortensen SA, et al. Early experience of double-lung transplantation with bronchial artery revascularization using mammary artery. Eur J Cardiothorac Surg 1994;8(10):520–4.

119. Pettersson G, Norgaard MA, Arendrup H, et al. Direct bronchial artery revascularization and en bloc double lung transplantation–surgical techniques and early outcome. J Heart Lung Transplant 1997;16(3):320–33.

120. Burton CM, Milman N, Carlsen J, et al. The Copenhagen National Lung Transplant Group: survival after single lung, double lung, and heart-lung transplantation. J Heart Lung Transplant 2005; 24(11):1834–43.

121. Schreinemakers HH, Weder W, Miyoshi S, et al. Direct revascularization of bronchial arteries for lung transplantation: an anatomical study. Ann Thorac Surg 1990;49(1):44–53 [discussion: 53–4].

122. Laks H, Louie HW, Haas GS, et al. New technique of vascularization of the trachea and bronchus for

lung transplantation. J Heart Lung Transplant 1991; 10(2):280–7.

123. Dubrez J, Clerc F, Drouillard J, et al. Anatomical bases for bronchial arterial revascularization in double lung transplantation. Ann Chir 1992;46(2):97–104.

124. Svendsen U, Arendrup H, Norgaard M, et al. Double lung transplantation with bronchial artery revascularization using mammary artery. Transplant Proc 1995;27(6):3485.

125. Norgaard MA, Olsen PS, Svendsen UG, et al. Revascularization of the bronchial arteries in lung transplantation: an overview. Ann Thorac Surg 1996;62(4):1215–21.

126. Pettersson G, Norgaard MA, Andersen CB, et al. Lung and heart-lung transplantation with direct bronchial artery revascularization. In: Hetzer R, editor. Lung transplantation. Darmstadt, Germany: Steinkopff Darmstadt; 1999.

127. Pettersson GB, Karam K, Thuita L, et al. Comparative study of bronchial artery revascularization in lung transplantation. J Thorac Cardiovasc Surg 2013;146(4):894–900.e3.

The Role of Bronchial Artery Revascularization in Lung Transplantation

Michael Z. Tong, MD, MBA[a,b], Douglas R. Johnston, MD[a,b],
Gosta B. Pettersson, MD, PhD[a,b],*

KEYWORDS

- Bronchial artery revascularization • Lung transplantation • Bronchiolitis obliterans syndrome
- Obliterative bronchiolitis

KEY POINTS

- Long-term survival of lung-transplant patients is 53% at 5 years and 31% at 10 years, which continues to lag behind the survival of other solid organs recipients.
- The modern era of lung transplantation has seen a shift from early mortality and complications related to the bronchial anastomosis to late mortality secondary to progressive organ dysfunction; the complex disease process may include elements of bronchiolitis obliterans syndrome, obliterative bronchiolitis, chronic rejection, or chronic lung allograft dysfunction.
- Although the initial goal of bronchial artery revascularization (BAR) was to reduce the incidence of airway ischemia and to improve bronchial healing, the benefits of restored bronchial artery circulation may extend beyond bronchial healing alone.
- Advantages of BAR include dramatically improving airway healing, decreasing airway complications, possibly better long-term survival compared with bilateral lung transplant, decreases in postoperative infection, less early rejection, and possibly delayed onset of progressive organ dysfunction.
- Disadvantages of BAR include being technically challenging, limited worldwide experience, extended surgical time and possibly ischemic time, increased risk of bleeding.

INTRODUCTION

The dual blood supply to the lungs consists of the pulmonary arterial tree and the small bronchial arteries (BAs). Although the bronchial circulation is known to be an important source of nutritive blood to the bronchial tree, most current techniques of lung transplantation do not restore the bronchial blood supply. Early in the clinical experience with lung transplantation, the primary barrier to clinical success, and the leading cause of mortality, was dehiscence or necrosis of the bronchial anastomosis.

The concept of bronchial artery revascularization (BAR) was known; however, the technically demanding nature of the procedure led surgeons to pursue alternative strategies to avoid bronchial complications. The lung transplant group at University of Toronto pioneered the method of wrapping the bronchial anastomosis with omentum,

Disclosures: The authors have nothing to disclose with regard to commercial support related to this topic.
[a] Department of Thoracic Surgery, Heart and Vascular Institute, Cleveland Clinic, 9500 Euclid Avenue, Cleveland, OH 44195, USA; [b] Department of Cardiovascular Surgery, Heart and Vascular Institute, Cleveland Clinic, 9500 Euclid Avenue, Cleveland, OH 44195, USA
* Corresponding author. Departments of Thoracic Surgery and Cardiovascular Surgery, Cleveland Clinic, 9500 Euclid Avenue, Mail Stop J4-1, Cleveland, OH 44195.
E-mail address: petterg@ccf.org

Thorac Surg Clin 25 (2015) 77–85
http://dx.doi.org/10.1016/j.thorsurg.2014.09.004
1547-4127/15/$ – see front matter © 2015 Elsevier Inc. All rights reserved.

which was demonstrated in animal studies to augment bronchial healing.[1,2] Subsequently, on November 7, 1983, Dr Joel Cooper performed the first successful single-lung transplantation on a 58-year-old Canadian dying of pulmonary fibrosis. In contrast to the success achieved in single-lung transplantation, en bloc double-lung transplantation (DLTX) performed with a tracheal anastomosis was plagued by a bronchial complication rate of 40%, even with omental wrapping.[3]

As a result of this experience, techniques for DLTX evolved to sequential implantation of the lungs with a very distal bronchial anastomosis at the hilum of the lung, with which wrapping was no longer necessary.[4] This technique was widely adopted by the lung transplant community, and DLTX performed en bloc was largely replaced with sequential bilateral lung transplantation (BLTX), and the interest in BAR waned. Unfortunately, bronchial ischemia and the resultant complications continued, albeit to a lesser extent. In the authors' practice, the bronchial complication rate remains in the 15% range, and in the current literature is between 3% and 25%.[5-12] Of note, there is emerging evidence that airway ischemia promotes airway fibrosis and *Aspergillus* invasion, and conversely, that improved microvascular circulation at the anastomosis site, mediated by exogenous angiogenesis promoting compounds, is able to attenuate this process.[13,14] Such studies add weight to the existing evidence that methods to promote normal airway perfusion and healing deserve ongoing attention from surgeons.

Direct BAR is the obvious solution to help ensure a normally healing and healthy airway. The technique was first described in dogs by Metras in 1950[15]; however, the first series of BA anastomoses in humans was not reported until the early 1990s by the group from Bordeaux, France in 1992, Harefield Hospital in United Kingdom in 1993, and Mayo Clinic, United States, and Copenhagen in 1994.[16-19] Although the early and midterm results of these studies were extremely favorable for bronchial healing, BAR did not gain wide acceptance in the lung transplant community secondary to increased technical difficulty, prolongation of ischemic and operative times, and increased risk of bleeding. In addition, most lung transplant programs were happy with their results using decreased steroid doses and distal bronchial anastomoses at the secondary carina. Consequently, en bloc DLTX was largely abandoned in favor of BLTX.

The modern era of lung transplantation has seen a shift from early mortality and complications related to the bronchial anastomosis to late mortality secondary to progressive organ dysfunction, the complex disease process that may include elements of bronchiolitis obliterans syndrome (BOS), obliterative bronchiolitis (OB), chronic rejection, or chronic lung allograft dysfunction.[20] Long-term survival remains close to 50% at 5 years, which is lower than that for other solid organ transplants. In 2005, long-term outcomes from the Copenhagen BAR series were published demonstrating excellent 5- and 10-year survival, superior to that of sequential lung transplant without BAR.[21] This article inspired one of the authors (G.B.P.) and the Cleveland Clinic lung transplant group to revisit BAR and to begin a pilot study to compare safety and efficacy compared with standard therapy and to study "teachability" of this more technically demanding procedure. The recent results are presented under "Long term results".

ANATOMY AND PHYSIOLOGY OF BRONCHIAL ARTERY SUPPLY

The BA circulation represents a small portion of the cardiac output, estimated to be 3% to 5% of total cardiac output during lung injury and inflammation, and perhaps less in the normal lung. It is considered important for airway defense, fluid balance, and lung metabolism because it delivers nutritive supply to airways, lung parenchyma, and lymph nodes and forms bronchopulmonary anastomoses along the alveoli.[22-24]

The anatomy of the BA is quite varied. Variations in bronchial arterial origin and course were well studied by Schreinemakers and colleagues[25] and have been confirmed by the authors' clinical experience with BAR.[26] The BAs, 1 to 4 in number, arise from the descending aorta and are among or medial to the upper right intercostal arteries (Fig. 1). The authors have previously described the anatomic variations and named the different arteries.[26] The most frequent and largest BA is the right intercostobronchial artery (RICBA), which arises as the first or second right intercostal artery and courses behind the esophagus, giving off the intercostal artery branch 1 to 2 cm after its origin from the aorta (Fig. 2). It then passes under the azygos vein and continues on the membranous portion of the right main bronchus. An RICBA can be found and secured in up to 90% of donor specimens according to Schreinemakers and colleagues.[25] In the authors' clinical experience, this figure is probably 75% to 80%. Left BAs have a direct route from the aorta to the left bronchus. It is unusual that no BA can be identified; this, however, may be the case when severe aortic atherosclerosis is present or when the BAs are inadvertently severed during harvest.

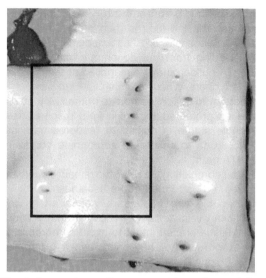

Fig. 1. Donor descending aorta with marking of the area within which BAs are originating. The first right intercostal branch ostium is usually the largest ostium and most likely to be the ostium of the RICBA. (*From* Pettersson GB, Yun JJ, Norgaard MA. Bronchial artery revascularization in lung transplantation: techniques, experience, and outcomes. Curr Opin Organ Transplant 2010;15(5):572–7; with permission.)

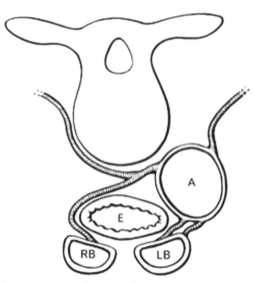

Fig. 2. Schematic drawing of the RICBA with its retro-esophageal course and 2 smaller left BAs. A, aorta; E, esophagus; LB, left bronchus; RB, right bronchus. (*Adapted from* Daly RC, McGregor CG. Routine immediate direct bronchial artery revascularization of bronchial arteries for single lung transplantation. Ann Thorac Surg 1994;57(6):1446–52; with permission.)

ORGAN HARVESTING, PRESERVATION, AND PREPARATION FOR BRONCHIAL ARTERY REVASCULARIZATION

Meticulous dissection in removal of the double lung block is essential to preserve continuity of the BAs. After cross-clamp, the heart and lungs are flushed and preserved. The heart is removed without violating the posterior pericardium. The pulmonary trunk is divided just above the pulmonary valve, leaving left and right pulmonary arteries in continuity with a short stump of main pulmonary artery. The pulmonary veins should be allowed a common cuff of left atrium. The trachea is stapled and divided as proximally as possible well above the level of the azygos vein. The esophagus is divided with a linear stapler proximally at the same level as the trachea and distally low in the chest. The lungs are removed en bloc with trachea, esophagus, and descending aorta. The esophagus has to be included to preserve the retroesophageal RICBA. It should be noted that the dissection must proceed very close to the chest wall, along the anterior aspect of the vertebral column so as not to injure the RICBA in its course behind the esophagus.

When the donor lung block arrives at the recipient operating room, the initial step in preparing the block is to carefully dissect the esophagus from the surrounding mediastinal tissue, leaving the retroesophageal tissue containing the RICBA intact. The aorta is opened longitudinally along its pleural surface opposite the origins of the intercostal and bronchial arteries. Inspection and gentle probing are used to identify the BAs. Most often, the RICBA immediately attracts attention as the first upper right and largest ostium among the intercostals (see **Figs. 1** and **2**). The RICBA is verified and the intercostal branch is localized and clipped; this is facilitated with the use of a small (1 mm) coronary probe. Left BAs, a BA trunk, or a carinal artery is found medial to the upper right intercostals.

If en bloc DLTX is intended, mediastinal tissue around the main bronchi, distal trachea, and carina is left intact. The pulmonary arteries are left in continuity for a pulmonary trunk anastomosis, and the pulmonary veins are prepared with cuffs of left atrium for bilateral left atrial anastomoses.

If a single-lung transplantation is intended, BAR is preferably performed for the lung with the most favorable anatomy. If both lungs are to be transplanted, securing good BAs to both lungs will be possible in less than 50% of the donor blocks.

SURGICAL IMPLANTATION TECHNIQUE FOR LUNG TRANSPLANTATION USING BRONCHIAL ARTERY REVASCULARIZATION

Choice of Conduit for Bronchial Artery Revascularization

The authors' preferred conduit is the internal thoracic artery (ITA) ("the mammary artery"), with early patency of 94%. The saphenous vein has been used by other groups but has lower patency.[27] The ITA (or vein) is harvested before arrival of the lungs. In the authors' institution, this is performed with skeletonized technique, which allows for maximal length and straightforward sequential anastomosis in the case of multiple BAs.

En Bloc Double Lung Transplantation with Bronchial Artery Revascularization

The surgeon cannot commit to en bloc transplantation until the donor block has been examined and useful BAs have been identified. En bloc DLTX is performed via sternotomy on cardiopulmonary bypass using standard aortic and bicaval cannulation. The left ITA is harvested before arrival of the donor lungs and left in situ. Cardiopulmonary bypass is initiated and dissection of both lung hila is carried out as would be routine for BLTX. In the case that the donor block is unfavorable for BAR, bronchial and PA anastomoses are performed in the standard fashion for BLTX. Once the donor block is confirmed as favorable for BAR, the trachea is divided by removing the main bronchi and carina, and dissection is carried out under the recipient left atrium to allow the donor block to be positioned appropriately. The main pulmonary artery is prepared and the pericardium is opened to a sufficient extent to allow the donor lung block to be introduced atraumatically.

Maintaining hemostasis is particularly important. Because the posterior dissection is more extensive than in the case of BLTX with more raw surface area, the authors find the use of an irrigated bipolar cautery (Aquamantys; Medtronic, Inc, Minneapolis, MN, USA) useful in achieving hemostasis before starting implantation. It is also important to think about minimizing contamination of the field by infectious material from the recipient airways. During introduction of the lung block, it is vital to verify the lungs are in the correct cavities and correctly oriented because it is possible for torsion of the block to occur at this stage. Iced slush is introduced to keep the lungs cold during the implantation. The left ITA to BA anastomoses are performed as the first anastomosis(-es), with the left lung and descending aorta of the donor block retracted from the left chest over the heart. Single or sequential anastomoses are performed

to the selected BA orifices using 7-0 Polypropylene sutures. The left lung is then replaced into the pleura. Successful BAR is immediately confirmed by bleeding from the donor mediastinal tissue. The ITA bulldog may be reapplied or the ITA may be left open. When returning the left lung, it is important to check the course of the ITA to make sure it is protected and not kinked. In some cases a single suture is placed to reapproximate the donor aorta to ensure an appropriate course of the ITA graft.

After completing the BAR, the remaining anastomoses are performed in the usual fashion for en bloc double lung: trachea, pulmonary artery, and pulmonary veins/left atria. Pericarinal and peribronchial tissue are left intact to avoid compromising the blood supply. The donor trachea is trimmed down to one ring above the carina. The pulmonary artery is anastomosed to the pulmonary trunk or to individual branches depending on what is available on the donor. The left atrial anastomoses are performed in the usual fashion for each side. En bloc DLTX with BAR can be performed in the same operative time as sequential BLTX without BAR (facilitated exposure and one tracheal anastomosis vs 2 bronchial anastomoses and 1 pulmonary artery vs 2 pulmonary artery anastomoses).

Single-Lung Transplantation with Bronchial Artery Revascularization

Single-lung transplantation is performed via lateral or anterior thoracotomy. The ITA is harvested before arrival of the donor lung. Explantation of the diseased lung and implantation of the donor lung are not different from routine single-lung transplant. However, the peribronchial tissue carrying the BAs must be preserved, leaving more of this tissue in place. A distal main bronchus anastomosis is performed as usual. Before reperfusion of the lung, 10,000 units of heparin are given. After the lung has been reperfused (pulmonary artery flow) and reventilated for a brief time, the ITA is divided. The lung is then dropped or gently ventilated while the BAR anastomosis is performed. The ITA harvest and the time it takes to perform the BAR anastomoses add 30 to 45 minutes to the overall duration of the operation, but do not add ischemic time.

OUTCOMES/RESULTS

Early Series

A human left single-lung transplantation including a BAR procedure was first attempted in 1973 by Dr Haglin and coworkers.[28] The patient died of infection after a few months but with a normally healing airway. The first human series of BAR was published by Couraud and coworkers[16] in Bordeaux, France in 1992, where they had performed 8 en bloc DLTX doing the BAR with saphenous vein grafts to the RICBA and left BAs. The distal anastomoses were done on the back table and the proximal anastomosis was performed at the end of the case. All patients had normal tracheal anastomosis healing, and bronchial arterial blood supply was visualized angiographically in 5 of the 7 patients. One patient died of pneumonia 1 month after surgery.

The following year, Sundset[29] from Harefield Hospital in London, United Kingdom presented 8 patients who underwent DLTX with BAR using the left ITA.[17,29] The BA was identified by probing with the largest vessel going in the direction of the carina chosen for revascularization. Seven patients had angiograms, which showed BA perfusion in 6, all of whom had normal airways. The one patient without BA supply developed a large ulcer at the tracheal anastomosis.

In 1994, Daly and colleagues[18] from the Mayo Clinic published a series of 10 patients with BAR in 10 single-lung transplant recipients. One patient died perioperatively of graft dysfunction. The remaining 9 had angiography demonstrating patent BAs in 7 and no perfusion in 2. Nevertheless, bronchial healing was excellent in all recipients. One interesting development in this series was the demonstration of the possibility of performing BAR on both lungs from the same donor by dividing the aorta between the left and right BAs.

In 1994, the Copenhagen group (G.B.P.) published a series of 14 en bloc with BAR using the left ITA, using the technique learned by G.B.P. from Sir Magdi Yacoub.[19] Ten were successful verified by angiography, whereas 2 were unsuccessful, both of whom developed left main bronchus stenosis ultimately requiring pneumonectomies. The next publication from Copenhagen included 47 en bloc DLTX with normal airway healing in 42, disturbed in 2, and complicated in 3. Angiographic BAR success rate was 94%. In the 3 patients with failed BAR, 2 required a pneumonectomy and 1 required retransplantation. In patients with successful BAR, 2-year patency of the IMA was 100%. The 1- and 2-year survival in this series was 83%. The G.B.P. Copenhagen series was later expanded to 68 DLTX, 1 BLTX, 27 single lung transplant, and 10 heart lung transplant with BAR, which still represents the largest experience with BAR in the world. There are other groups who have performed smaller numbers of lung transplants with BAR.

The authors know from personal communication, 2014, that Dr Dean McKenzie in Houston has performed several en bloc DLTX in children wherein he has directly implanted the BAs with an aortic button in the descending aorta with good outcomes, and they are eager to see longer-term data from those patients.

Long-term Results

Few long-term data exist regarding the effect of BAR on patient survival or graft-related complications. Norgaard and colleagues[30] later evaluated the long-term results of their first 62 en bloc DLTX and found 1-, 2-, 3-, 4-, and 5-year survivals to be 85%, 81%, 69%, 69%, and 69%, respectively.[30] Patients who had complete or incomplete bilateral BAR had better survival versus incomplete hemilateral, incomplete poor, or failed BAR. Compared with a control group from Stanford who performed sequential BLTX, the onset of BOS and OB appeared to be delayed in the BAR patients, although no formal statistics were performed (**Fig. 3**). Of interest, in patients surviving 3 months or more after transplant, the postoperative baseline forced expiratory volume in 1 second was lower in patients who later developed BOS or OB, suggesting that the process that leads to BOS and OB may start early. Therefore, if BAR can lead to delayed BOS and OB, it appeared possible that BAR may prolong survival. This long-term survival advantage was demonstrated in the results published by the Copenhagen National Lung Transplant Group in which 5-year survival for en bloc DLTX with BAR was 69% versus 57% for the sequential DLTX group, although the cohorts were not matched.[21]

As a result of the positive long-term results demonstrated in the Copenhagen series, there was renewed interest in BAR. Based on the extensive BAR experience of one of the authors (G.B.P.), a pilot study was undertaken at the Cleveland Clinic to demonstrate (1) whether the results of the Copenhagen series could be repeated and were favorable to existing techniques and (2) whether the Copenhagen BAR technique could be generalized to other surgeons. To date, 37 lung transplants with BAR have been performed at the Cleveland Clinic. The first 27 were published in a single-center, nonrandomized, 1:2 propensity matched study comparing 27 BAR patients to 54 routine non-BAR patients.[31] BAR and non-BAR patients had similar cardiopulmonary bypass (CPB) time, skin-to-skin time, intensive care unit (ICU) length of stay (LOS), postoperative LOS, requirement for tracheostomy, and extracorporeal membrane oxygenation (ECMO). Bleeding requiring reintervention was higher in the BAR group, 37% versus 9.3% (**Table 1**). Twenty-four of 25 BAR patients demonstrated a patent IMA

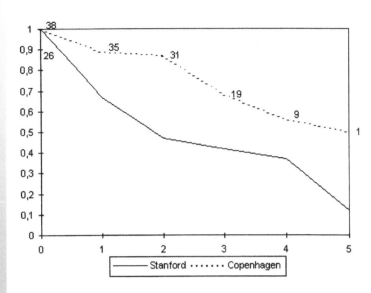

Fig. 3. A comparison of freedom from BOS after lung transplantation between Copenhagen (en bloc DLTX) and Stanford (BLTX). (*From* Norgaard MA, Andersen CB, Pettersson G. Does bronchial artery revascularization influence results concerning bronchiolitis obliterans syndrome and/or obliterative bronchiolitis after lung transplantation? Eur J Cardiothorac Surg 1998;14(3):311–8; with permission.)

and BA. One patient with normal airway healing declined angiogram. One patient died 6 weeks after transplantation and before imaging; however, autopsy showed a patent BAR and normal healing airways.

As expected, the incidence of airway ischemia was significantly lower in the BAR group of 3.7%, compared with the non-BAR group of 22%.

Among the 12 non-BAR patients with airway complications, 8 required airway intervention, including 3 balloon bronchial dilatations and 5 multiple and complex interventions, including airway stenting. The incidence of PGD was not different between the groups. In the first 3 months, the incidence of rejection was lower in the BAR group, but no difference was found beyond the initial 3 months.

Table 1
Safety and efficacy data from the comparative study of bronchial artery revascularization in lung transplantation

	BAR (n = 27)	Non BAR (n = 54)	
Safety			
CPB times	164 ± 32	178 ± 78	$P = .3$
Skin-to-skin time	350 ± 71	318 ± 86	$P = .07$
ICU stay 15th/median/85th percentile	3/7/23	2/5/21	$P = .16$
Postoperative stay 15th/median/85th percentile	10/19/57	8/15/31	$P = .2$
Reoperation for bleeding	10 (37%)	5 (9.3%)	$P = .002$
Tracheostomy	9	10	$P = .2$
ECMO	1	4	$P = .07$
Clinical effectiveness			
Airway ischemia	1 (3.7%)	12 (22%)	$P = .03$
Rejection <3 mo (freedom from rejection)	77%	57%	$P = .08$
Rejection >3 mo			NS
Primary graft dysfunction (PGD)			NS
Infection within 1 y (events/100 patient-years)	30	58	$P = .04$
Bloodstream infections	2	19	
Survival 1/3/6 mo/1/2 y (%)	100/96/96/96/83	96/96/93/90/80	$P = .6$

From Pettersson GB, Karam K, Thuita L, et al. Comparative study of bronchial artery revascularization in lung transplantation. J Thorac Cardiovasc Surg 2013;146(4):894–900.e3; with permission.

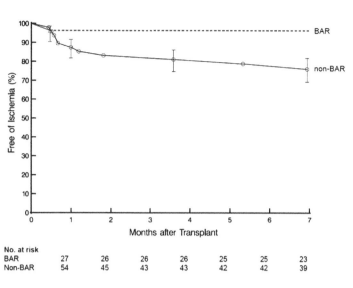

Fig. 4. Freedom form airway ischemia. (*From* Pettersson GB, Karam K, Thuita L, et al. Comparative study of bronchial artery revascularization in lung transplantation. J Thorac Cardiovasc Surg 2013;146(4):894–900.e3; with permission.)

Pulmonary infection was also significantly lower in the BAR group, 30 per 100 patient-years versus 58 per 100 patient-years. The incidence of blood-stream infections was also significantly lower in favor of BAR. Freedom from BOS at 24 months also trended to favor BAR at 92% versus58%; however, this difference was not statistically significant ($P = .07-.14$). Mortality between the groups is similar up to 2 years. The figures from **Figs. 4–6** are taken from the authors' most recent publication.[31]

DISCUSSION

Clinical outcomes after lung transplantation have improved since the late 1980s, but overall survival still trails that of other solid organs, currently at 53% at 5 years and 31% at 10 years.[32] BOS and infection are responsible for approximately 50% of the total mortality at 5 years.[32] Although the incidence of early airway complications has improved with decreased steroid dosage and resection of most of the extrapulmonary main bronchi, these serious complications still occur in about 15% of cases. BOS and OB remain a significant problem for long-term durability of the organ and for patient survival. There is some evidence that the process that leads to BOS and OB seems to start very early and may be related to acute rejection and ischemia.[13]

Although the initial goal of BAR was to reduce the incidence of airway ischemia and to improve bronchial healing, the benefits of restored BA circulation may extend beyond bronchial healing alone. In both the Copenhagen and the Cleveland Clinic experience, there appears to be multiple

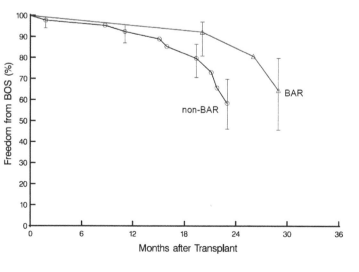

Fig. 5. Freedom from BOS. (*From* Pettersson GB, Karam K, Thuita L, et al. Comparative study of bronchial artery revascularization in lung transplantation. J Thorac Cardiovasc Surg 2013;146(4):894–900.e3; with permission.)

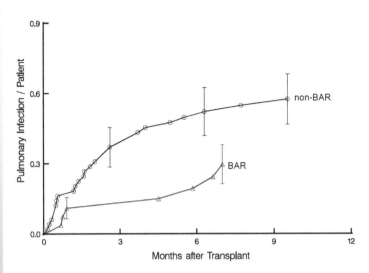

Fig. 6. Pulmonary infections after transplant. (*From* Pettersson GB, Karam K, Thuita L, et al. Comparative study of bronchial artery revascularization in lung transplantation. J Thorac Cardiovasc Surg 2013;146(4):894–900.e3; with permission.)

benefits of BAR. That patients with BAR had fewer infections, suggests that physiologic BA supply may restore a more normal regulation of inflammation, fluid balance, and airway defense. Of additional importance is the finding that BAR impacts not only early rejection but also potentially the long-term incidence of BOS. These factors may partly explain why the early Copenhagen series of en bloc DLTX with BAR had a 5-year survival of 69%, which is better than contemporary results with BLTX.

To date, the barrier to larger adoption of BAR has been the increased technical complexity and time. The current Cleveland Clinic BAR study attempts to address the issue of generalizability or "teachability." Although this phase of the study is ongoing, it should be noted that all BAR procedures performed by 2 surgeons other than the study originator (G.B.P.) have been successful.

REFERENCES

1. Lima O, Goldberg M, Peters WJ, et al. Bronchial omentopexy in canine lung transplantation. J Thorac Cardiovasc Surg 1982;83(3):418–21.
2. Morgan E, Lima O, Goldberg M, et al. Improved bronchial healing in canine left lung reimplantation using omental pedicle wrap. J Thorac Cardiovasc Surg 1983;85(1):134–9.
3. Patterson GA, Todd TR, Cooper JD, et al. Airway complications after double lung transplantation. Toronto Lung Transplant Group. J Thorac Cardiovasc Surg 1990;99(1):14–20 [discussion: 20–1].
4. Patterson GA. Airway revascularization: is it necessary? Ann Thorac Surg 1993;56(4):807–8.
5. Date H, Trulock EP, Arcidi JM, et al. Improved airway healing after lung transplantation. An analysis of 348 bronchial anastomoses. J Thorac Cardiovasc Surg 1995;110(5):1424–32 [discussion: 1432–3].
6. Ruttmann E, Ulmer H, Marchese M, et al. Evaluation of factors damaging the bronchial wall in lung transplantation. J Heart Lung Transplant 2005; 24(3):275–81.
7. Schroder C, Scholl F, Daon E, et al. A modified bronchial anastomosis technique for lung transplantation. Ann Thorac Surg 2003;75(6):1697–704.
8. Choong CK, Sweet SC, Zoole JB, et al. Bronchial airway anastomotic complications after pediatric lung transplantation: Incidence, cause, management, and outcome. J Thorac Cardiovasc Surg 2006;131(1):198–203.
9. Herrera JM, McNeil KD, Higgins RS, et al. Airway complications after lung transplantation: treatment and long-term outcome. Ann Thorac Surg 2001; 71(3):989–93 [discussion: 993–4].
10. Aigner C, Jaksch P, Seebacher G, et al. Single running suture–the new standard technique for bronchial anastomoses in lung transplantation. Eur J Cardiothorac Surg 2003;23(4):488–93.
11. Murthy SC, Blackstone EH, Gildea TR, et al. Impact of anastomotic airway complications after lung transplantation. Ann Thorac Surg 2007; 84(2):401–9, 409.e1–4.
12. Van De Wauwer C, Van Raemdonck D, Verleden GM, et al. Risk factors for airway complications within the first year after lung transplantation. Eur J Cardiothorac Surg 2007;31(4):703–10.
13. Nicolls MR, Zamora MR. Bronchial blood supply after lung transplantation without bronchial artery revascularization. Curr Opin Organ Transplant 2010;15(5):563–7.
14. Dhillon GS, Zamora MR, Roos JE, et al. Lung transplant airway hypoxia: a diathesis to fibrosis? Am J Respir Crit Care Med 2010;182(2):230–6.

15. Metras H. Note preliminaire sur la greffe du total du poumon chez le chien. Proc Acad Sci 1950;231: 1176–7.
16. Couraud L, Baudet E, Nashef SA, et al. Lung transplantation with bronchial revascularisation. Surgical anatomy, operative technique and early results. Eur J Cardiothorac Surg 1992;6(9):490–5.
17. Daly RC, Tadjkarimi S, Khaghani A, et al. Successful double-lung transplantation with direct bronchial artery revascularization. Ann Thorac Surg 1993; 56(4):885–92.
18. Daly RC, McGregor CG. Routine immediate direct bronchial artery revascularization for single-lung transplantation. Ann Thorac Surg 1994;57(6): 1446–52.
19. Pettersson G, Arendrup H, Mortensen SA, et al. Early experience of double-lung transplantation with bronchial artery revascularization using mammary artery. Eur J Cardiothorac Surg 1994;8(10): 520–4.
20. Verleden GM, Raghu G, Meyer KC, et al. A new classification system for chronic lung allograft dysfunction. J Heart Lung Transplant 2014;33(2):127–33.
21. Burton CM, Milman N, Carlsen J, et al. The Copenhagen National Lung Transplant Group: survival after single lung, double lung, and heart-lung transplantation. J Heart Lung Transplant 2005;24(11): 1834–43.
22. Wagner EM, Foster WM. Importance of airway blood flow on particle clearance from the lung. J Appl Physiol (1985) 1996;81(5):1878–83.
23. Wagner EM, Blosser S, Mitzner W. Bronchial vascular contribution to lung lymph flow. J Appl Physiol (1985) 1998;85(6):2190–5.
24. Deffebach ME, Charan NB, Lakshminarayan S, et al. The bronchial circulation. Small, but a vital attribute of the lung. Am Rev Respir Dis 1987; 135(2):463–81.
25. Schreinemakers HH, Weder W, Miyoshi S, et al. Direct revascularization of bronchial arteries for lung transplantation: an anatomical study. Ann Thorac Surg 1990;49(1):44–53 [discussion: 53–4].
26. Pettersson GB, Yun JJ, Norgaard MA. Bronchial artery revascularization in lung transplantation: techniques, experience, and outcomes. Curr Opin Organ Transplant 2010;15(5):572–7.
27. Norgaard MA, Efsen F, Arendrup H, et al. Surgical and arteriographic results of bronchial artery revascularization in lung and heart lung transplantation. J Heart Lung Transplant 1997;16(3):302–12.
28. Haglin JJ, Ruiz E, Baker RC, et al. Histologic studies of human lung allotransplantation. Basel (Switzerland): S. Karger; 1973.
29. Sundset A, Tadjkarimi S, Khaghani A, et al. Human en bloc double-lung transplantation: bronchial artery revascularization improves airway perfusion. Ann Thorac Surg 1997;63(3):790–5.
30. Norgaard MA, Andersen CB, Pettersson G. Does bronchial artery revascularization influence results concerning bronchiolitis obliterans syndrome and/ or obliterative bronchiolitis after lung transplantation? Eur J Cardiothorac Surg 1998;14(3):311–8.
31. Pettersson GB, Karam K, Thuita L, et al. Comparative study of bronchial artery revascularization in lung transplantation. J Thorac Cardiovasc Surg 2013;146(4):894–900.e3.
32. Yusen RD, Christie JD, Edwards LB, et al. The Registry of the International Society for Heart and Lung Transplantation: Thirtieth Adult Lung and Heart-Lung Transplant Report–2013; focus theme: age. J Heart Lung Transplant 2013; 32(10):965–78.

Pleural Space Complications Associated with Lung Transplantation

Andrew Arndt, MD, Daniel J. Boffa, MD*

KEYWORDS

- Lung transplantation • Pleural space complications • Hemothorax • Chylothorax

KEY POINTS

- Despite decreasing operative mortality, lung transplantation continues to carry significant risk of pleural space complications.
- In addition to addressing pleural space disease, it is important to evaluate for other complications that could be driving the pleural process (eg, rejection, bronchopleural fistula, pulmonary vein stenosis).
- Pleural space complications are associated with a compromise in short-term survival. Therefore, attempts should be made to prevent pleural space complications and minimize their impact should they develop.

INTRODUCTION

Lung transplantation represents a life-saving option for a variety of end-stage lung diseases. Despite the magnitude of anatomic manipulation and the fragility of the patient population, the procedures have become progressively safer over time, with operative mortalities decreasing from 19% to 10% over the past 2 decades.[1–3] Perioperative morbidity, however, remains high. Pleural space complications are particularly common, occurring in 22% to 34% of patients.[4,5] Pleural complications include a constellation of hemorrhagic, infectious, inflammatory, or other processes that result in the accumulation of fluid, debris, and air within the pleural space. The impact on pleural complications on allograft function and overall patient recovery can be significant, particularly in the setting of persistently borderline cardiopulmonary reserve. Although surgeons have greatly advanced the care of pleural space complications in the general thoracic patient population, lung transplant recipients are typically more fragile and their postoperative course is generally more tenuous than most general thoracic patients. In addition, the need for immunosuppression renders the management of pleural complications particularly challenging in this population.

OVERVIEW OF POSTTRANSPLANT PLEURAL SPACE COMPLICATIONS

Several factors predispose lung transplant recipients to the development of pleural space complications, perhaps most notably pleural space abnormalities that predate the transplant. For example, the pathologic conditions responsible for the end-stage lung disease can often result in infectious or inflammatory changes in the pleural space. Furthermore, procedures to diagnose the end-stage lung disease (ie, wedge biopsy), as well as procedures to treat complications of end-stage lung disease (eg, pleurodesis for pneumothorax), may result in the fusion of the visceral and parietal pleura. Explanation of the diseased lungs in the setting of pleural symphysis can result

Disclosures: None.
Thoracic Surgery, Yale New Haven Hospital, New Heaven, CT 06510, USA
* Corresponding author.
E-mail address: daniel.boffa@yale.edu

Thorac Surg Clin 25 (2015) 87–95
http://dx.doi.org/10.1016/j.thorsurg.2014.09.005

in significant trauma to the soft tissue of the inner chest cavity (increasing risk of postoperative hemorrhage), as well as spillage of contaminated material from the diseased lung into the pleural space (increasing risk of pleural space infections). One surgical series noted pleural alteration in 54% of patients preoperatively (pleural thickening, most commonly, but also calcification, pneumothorax, and pleural effusion).[5] For the sake of this article, pleural complications are organized into following categories: hemothorax, chylothorax, air leak or pneumothorax, recurrent effusion, empyema, trapped lung, and chronic pleural complications (fibrothorax).

Hemothorax

The accumulation of a hemothorax after lung transplantation is concerning for both active blood loss, as well as pleural space complication. The merits of blood conservation seem to apply to nearly every category of major surgical procedures; therefore, early reoperation to minimize blood transfusion after lung transplantation is justifiable. The surgeon must balance the risks of reoperation with the probability of spontaneous cessation as well as the likelihood of finding a surgically addressable source (as opposed to diffuse chest wall oozing or bleeding that reflects an incompletely corrected coagulopathy). To this end, several steps can be taken to minimize the risks of perioperative bleeding. The raw surface oozing often reflects vascular adhesions between the native lung and chest wall. Although a meticulous dissection at the time of pulmonary explant must be balanced against ischemia time for the allograft, a dissection does not have to be slow to be hemostatic. Blunt dissection should be avoided in areas of vascular adhesions, in favor of cautery. In areas of particularly dense adhesions, the LigaSure (Covidien, Norwalk, CT) can be useful, or stapling off a slip of adherent lung (and potentially returning to this area to excise residual native lung once the lung has been removed or after the new lung has been placed). If the patient is going to go on cardiopulmonary bypass, it is advisable to dissect the native lung and obtain hemostasis before fully anticoagulating. On completion of anastomoses, persistent raw surface oozing can be addressed using the argon beam coagulator. Early recognition of the potential need for this step can save several minutes at the end of the case waiting for the Argon beam to be set up. Raw surface oozing may also be addressed by applying topical hemostatic agents, such as Surgicel, Gelfoam or thrombin, Surgiflo, Floseal, and other agents. There are little

published data on the safety of using these agents around a transplanted lung, and they likely have a similar risk profile as in the general thoracic population. If the patient is perceived to be at particular risk for oozing, it would be worth ensuring the chest is adequately drained with large-bore chest tubes, in hopes of preventing the accumulation of clotted blood (see later discussion).

Residual hemothorax (not associated with active blood loss) is identified in up to 15% of lung transplant recipients, potentially being more common when cardiopulmonary bypass is used.[4,5] Retained blood in the pleural space could extrinsically compromise ventilation of the transplanted lung as well as serve as a nidus for infection or potentially lead to chronic pleural space complications (eg, trapped lung, fibrothorax). Hospital mortality seems to be higher in patients that develop hemothorax, but it is difficult to isolate this outcome variable as the sole driver of operative mortality.[5,6]

Evacuation of a hemothorax can be attempted by large-bore tube thoracostomy, yet the blood is often clotted and does not drain well. However, safe and successful instillation of thrombolytics has been described in the transplant population.[7] In the event of failure of tube thoracostomy and thrombolytics, reoperation to evacuate a residual hemothorax can often be accomplished safely by video-assisted thoracoscopic surgery (VATS).

Chylothorax

Chylothorax is an infrequent complication following lung transplantation, occurring in less than 1% of lung transplant recipients.[4,5] The diagnosis of chylothorax generally requires the patient to be undergoing enteric feeding and is suggested by a transition to milky colored pleural effluent. The presence of chylomicrons or a triglyceride level greater than 110 mg/dL in the pleural fluid is diagnostic for chylothorax.[8] The consequences of chylothorax among lung transplant patients mirror those in other patients and include malnutrition, electrolyte abnormalities, and immune suppression from the ongoing loss of lymphatic fluid.[9] The immunosuppressive effects are of particular importance in this population and may lead to a need for immunosuppressant dose adjustment.[10]

Typically a trial of bowel rest is initiated to evaluate for spontaneous resolution of chyle leak. During this time period the patient may require total parenteral nutrition (TPN) for nutritional support, depending on the duration of bowel rest. Despite the known immunosuppressive effects of TPN,[11] it has been used without apparent adverse results in lung transplant patients.[9] Other nutritional support options include modified enteric feeds (alimental formula with no fats or medium-chain triglyceride diet). A determination of success or failure of a bowel rest approach should be rendered within 10 to 14 days to avoid prolonged depletion from ongoing lymph drainage. Pleurodesis may be attempted in the setting of low output, but the efficacy suffers from the steroid-impaired inflammatory response. Attempts to eliminate depletion by recirculating the lymph fluid (ie, pleuroperitoneal or pleurovenous shunts) would be reserved for patients in whom thoracic duct ligation was too high risk or not possible.

Thoracic duct ligation is a highly effective means to resolve a chylothorax but requires a secondary operation. This is typically approached from the right hemithorax by encircling the soft tissue between the aorta and lateral border of the azygous vein in the distal chest cavity. Unless there was an unusual degree of manipulation at the level of the hiatus, the surgeon should prioritize a safe, less traumatic passage of a suture or tie in the distal chest, rather than trying to ligate the absolute lowest point of the thoracic course of the thoracic duct (as is done for esophagectomy-associated chylothoraces). This ligation can be done by VATS.

Surgical ligation of the thoracic duct can at times be problematic in the setting of a fresh lung transplant. For example lung isolation (bronchial blocker, double-lumen endotracheal tube) may traumatize a fresh airway anastomosis. A patient recovering from a single lung transplant on the right side may not tolerate right lung isolation. The VATS approach with CO_2 insufflation may eliminate the need for total lung isolation. The thoracic duct can also be ligated transabdominally via laparoscopy.

More recently, thoracic duct embolization has represented another therapeutic option in transplant patients with chylothorax. Its main advantages include avoidance of reoperation and avoidance of general anesthesia. The procedure entails performing a lymphangiogram via injection of isosulfan blue in a pedal lymphatic followed by right posterior transhepatic cannulation of the cisterna chyli once radiographically opacified. The identified cisterna chyli is then embolized with cyanoacrylate "glue" or metallic embolization coils. This procedure has proven to be both safe and effective.[12]

Prolonged Air Leak

In contrast to transient air leak, prolonged air leak following lung transplantation can be problematic, contributing to prolonged length of stay and potentially to pleural space infections. Because most donors are younger and healthier, air leaks would be expected to occur less frequently than in patients undergoing pulmonary surgery in the setting of emphysematous disease. Indeed any significant air leak should at least raise the question of possible breakdown at the bronchial anastomosis and should prompt the consideration of flexible bronchoscopy. However, several processes can occur in the transplanted lung that can contribute to parenchymal injury resulting in air extravasation, including infection, rejection, and possibly ischemia from loss of bronchial arterial circulation.[5]

The prevalence has been reported by smaller series to range from 1% to 10%.[4,5] On both univariate and multivariate analysis, prolonged air leak was associated with an increased risk of postoperative death ($P = .02$ and $P = .011$, respectively).[5]

The use of split lung transplants between living donors represents a further source of air leak from the parenchymal suture line. If the suture-line appears to be leaking at the time of transplantation, the surgeon can attempt to address this via oversewing of any portion of a dehisced staple line if present. The use of topical sealants has not been used widely enough in this population to make any generalization concerning their safety or efficacy. In general, it is not advisable to place a sealant near a bronchial anastomosis because this may potentially be associated with infectious and healing complications at this level.

Recurrent Pleural Effusions

Lung transplantation is associated with varying degrees of postoperative pleural fluid production necessitating the use of pleural drains. There is at least some indication that the volume of pleural drainage and the duration that chest tubes remain in place are greater in transplant recipients than other types of thoracic surgery.[5] Possible mechanisms for the postoperative fluid drainage include increased alveolar capillary permeability,[13] temporary disruption of lymphatic drainage (which ultimately reconstitutes),[14] acute rejection,[15] or early overhydration.[5] There seems to be considerable variability between patients (eg, one study reported a mean duration of tube thoracostomy drainage 19.4 days with a range of 5–52 days).[5] Prolonged or particularly voluminous chest drain effluent should prompt an evaluation for other associated pathologic conditions, such as a thoracic duct leak (typically obvious from the character of the fluid), or pulmonary vein stenosis (typically associated with a more broadly abnormal clinical picture, such as new or worsened dyspnea, cough, or hemoptysis).[16]

Recurrent pleural effusions (those that develop after the removal of the pleural drains) can be more problematic because the associated atelectasis may compromise function of the allograft, lead to pneumonias in hypoventilated lung, become secondarily infected, or develop into chronic pleural space complications (ie, trapped lung).

In a series in which chest tubes were routinely removed within 7 days postoperatively, subsequent effusions developed in 124 of 455 patients (27%).[17] Traditional maneuvers to alleviate perioperative pleural effusions such as diuresis, thoracentesis, or surveillance for spontaneous resorbtion are reasonable. Marom and colleagues[7] presented a series of 214 lung transplant recipients, of whom 31 (14%) underwent temporary small-bore catheter drainage of pleural effusions. The indication for drainage varied and included parapneumonic effusion,[10] empyema,[6] rejection, and other causes of pleural fluid accumulation.[8] Time from transplantation to drainage ranged from 5 days to 36 months, with a median time of 1.8 months. Response to drainage was evaluated immediately after catheter insertion and at 30 and 90 days following catheter removal. At each point in time, respectively, only 5%, 6%, and 4% of patients available for follow-up did not experience either a complete or at least partial response (smaller effusion radiographically than that seen on preprocedural imaging). However, the authors note that many patients required multiple drainage procedures or lytic therapy with streptokinase. No mention is made of complications associated with instillation of streptokinase. Additionally, the authors note that in 12 study subjects who did not undergo drainage of a contralateral effusion, only 2 of 12 effusions were not at least partially resolved at the 90-day reimaging, suggesting that many of the effusions may have improved without intervention.[7]

However, a subset of patients will develop recurrent pleural effusions that persist despite these perioperative management strategies. In addition, pleural effusions can become loculated, precluding simple drainage. Clinicians must balance the risk of secondary procedures and prolonged chest drainage with the estimated consequences of allowing the effusion to remain. Reoperation with pleurodesis is a reasonable approach in patients with recurrent pleural effusions and may be accomplished via VATS. The surgeon must assess whether there is sufficient apposition between visceral and parietal pleura to perform the pleurodesis. It is important to note that, although pleurodesis has been described in the lung transplant population, concurrent steroid use markedly inhibits the inflammatory response and has been shown to dramatically reduce the efficacy of both talc and doxycycline pleurodesis.[18,19] Additionally, pleurodesis via tube thoracostomy has been reported to incite empyema in immunosuppressed patients.[20] That being said, it is not an unreasonable maneuver if the clinical picture warrants this step.

If the lung is trapped, a decortication (see later discussion) may be performed or, alternatively, a chronic drainage catheter could be placed. Surgical decortication for loculated pleural effusion was performed in 7 lung transplant recipients at the Cleveland Clinic between 1990 and 2006 (1.3%).[6] Complete lung re-expansion was identified in 5 subjects (71%) and 1 (14%) subject died during the hospitalization. In the Cleveland Clinic series, the longitudinal outcomes were reported for sbjects undergoing decortication of a transplanted lung (loculated effusion 7, empyema 15, hemothorax 3, and fibrothorax 2) (**Fig. 1**).

Chronic drainage via tunneled catheters is also a reasonable choice for patients in whom pleurodesis has failed or patients with a trapped lung who are unable to tolerate a decortication. The use of tunneled catheters has been recently

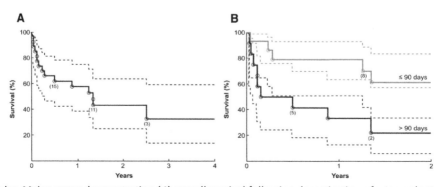

Fig. 1. Kaplan-Meier curves demonstrating (*A*) overall survival following decortication of a transplanted lung and (*B*) the significantly improved survival of those undergoing decortication within 90-days posttransplant (CI, *dashed lines*). (*From* Boffa DJ, Mason DP, Su JW, et al. Decortication after lung transplantation. Ann Thorac Surg 2008;85:1041; with permission.)

described for the management of posttransplant effusions. The first such series reported the outcomes of 12 PleurX insertions for pleural effusion refractory to thoracentesis or tube thoracostomy. Eight of the 12 effusions (67%) were also associated with entrapped lungs. All patients selected for this management strategy were considered poor candidates for decortication or thought to have a degree of entrapment amenable to less invasive treatment. Eleven of the 12 catheter placements resulted in complete lung re-expansion, whereas only 1 of 12 ultimately required decortication for empyema. One patient on anticoagulation who developed hemothorax following catheter insertion was successfully treated with thrombolytic instillation. Median catheter duration was 86 days.[21] This study, though small, suggests that pleurocutaneous catheter insertion is a safe and effective technique for the management of pleural space complications following lung transplantation.

Empyema, Trapped Lung, Fibrothorax

Empyema can represent a particularly challenging complication after lung transplantation. Infected fluid or debris in the pleural space may serve as a source for systemic infection in the immunocompromised lung transplant recipient and must be addressed aggressively. Empyema has been reported to occur in 3% to 8% of lung transplant recipients.[4,5,17,22] Although empyema was originally reported to occur significantly more often following double-lung transplants,[4] subsequent reports found no difference in the rate of empyema based on the type of transplant (single-lung, double-lung, heart-lung).[22] Wahidi and colleagues[17] did affirm a trend toward association with double-lung transplant over single-lung transplant ($P = .06$) but, ultimately, concluded that no patient demographic or preoperative factors were significantly associated with an increased risk of empyema. Interestingly, cystic fibrosis (CF) patients, in whom colonization with infectious pulmonary pathogens is the norm, do not seem to be at increased risk for pleural space infections after lung transplant.[22]

The clinical presentation of empyema may be somewhat less impressive than in the general thoracic population because the typical signs and symptoms may be blunted by immunosuppression. Radiographic findings may resemble residual noninfectious processes such as hemothorax or recurrent pleural effusions. In addition, pleural effluent after lung transplantation commonly has the biochemical profile of an empyema, even if sterile (ie, 96% of patients will meet

Light's criteria for empyema in the pleural drainage), making the diagnosis challenging to establish. Pleural fluid analysis can nonetheless be quite useful. In contrast to noninfected effusions, infected effusions have a statistically significantly higher l-lactate dehydrogenase (LDH) and neutrophil count as well as a lower lymphocyte count. Applying a cutoff of pleural fluid neutrophils greater than 21% yields a sensitivity of 70% and specificity of 79% for correctly identifying infected versus noninfected pleural effusion.[17] Preoperative colonization has been presumed to be a causative factor in the development of posttransplant empyema; however, the presentation is often delayed for a mean of 6 weeks, which is a bit longer than would be expected for this mechanism. It is likely that the pleural space is secondarily infected by transient bacteremia or fungemia associated with other soft tissue infections or peripheral or central vascular access infections.[22]

Empyema is typically monomicrobial (71.4%) but may be polymicrobial (14.3%) or have no organism isolated (14.3%).[22] Fungal pathogens are rather frequently encountered (61% of the time), with *Candida albicans* being the most common of these. Gram-negative bacteria cause 25% of posttransplant empyema. Other atypical causes include *Mycoplasma* and *Mycobacterium tuberculosis*. The high rate of fungus identification in this cohort may be secondary to routine obtaining of fungal cultures in all posttransplant effusions as well as the combination of immunosuppression and bacterial prophylaxis suppressing bacterial growth while allowing fungal proliferation.[17]

Prompt recognition and treatment of empyema is critical because empyema portends increased morbidity and mortality. It has been found to be associated with increased risk of postoperative death on univariate analysis ($P = .05$).[5] In a study by Nunley and colleagues,[22] 28.6% of empyema subjects died. Ferrer and colleagues[5] reported death in 2 of 3 empyema subjects (both with *Aspergillus* infection). The lone survivor required permanent pleural drainage for an *Acinetobacter* pleural infection. In another study, empyema was found to be the only pleural complication associated with death.[4] In the series reported by Wahidi and colleagues,[17] the 1-year survival was 86% if no effusion present, 91% if sterile effusion present, and 67% if empyema occurred. Survival was statistically lower for the empyema group compared with the noninfection group (87% 1-year survival) overall ($P = .002$). Death was caused by sepsis and subsequent multiple organ system failure 82% of time. In 67% of sepsis deaths, the blood pathogen is identical to the pleural fluid pathogen.[17]

Once diagnosed, the management of posttransplant empyema includes both the appropriate antibiotics for the offending organism and evacuation of the infected fluid and debris from the pleural space. The evacuation procedure can vary based on the type of material in the space. For empyemas in the early or inflammatory phase, the predominately free-flowing fluid can be drained via thoracentesis. For empyemas in the fibrinopurulent phase, the mixture of fluid, gelatinous material, and purulence can be addressed with a chest tube, a chest tube with instilled fibrinolytic agents, or a surgical decortication.

Once an empyema has reached the fibrotic phase, a decortication is the most definitive option provided that the patient will tolerate it. In one series regarding posttransplant empyema, 17% were managed with thoracentesis, 67% with chest tube drainage, and 17% with surgical decortication.[17] Another series reports surgical decortication having been performed for empyema in 15 subjects (2.7% of lung transplants) over a 15-year period at the Cleveland Clinic.[6] The hospital mortality was particularly high for subjects undergoing decortication for empyema at 40%. In this series, decortication overall was performed 27 times in 24 of the 553 subjects (4.3%). The general indications for decortication were pleural thickening with associated lung entrapment seen on computed tomography and loculated fluid collections not amenable to percutaneous drainage. Empyema was the most common specific indication for decortication (15 of 27 cases). Other posttransplant complications requiring decortication included loculated effusion (7 of 27), hemothorax (3 of 27), and fibrothorax (2 of 27).[6]

The operative approach for decortication was most typically posterolateral thoracotomy,[22] with other surgical options being VATS (3), redo clamshell (1), and sternotomy (1). The procedure was performed with an initial extrapleural dissection that culminated in complete parietal and visceral decortications until the achievement of maximal lung re-expansion (**Fig. 2**).[6]

Decortication timing ranged from 12 days to 7.8 years postoperatively, with a median time of 81 days. The 3 VATS decortications occurred at a median time of 25 days postoperatively, whereas the open decortications occurred with a median time of 82 days postoperatively, with the difference in timing reflecting prior attempts at more conservative drainage procedures in the open decortication group as well as that the decortication performed earlier likely addressed the pleural complication at a less organized stage, allowing a more minimally invasive approach.[6] This finding is concordant with other reports of thoracoscopic decortications for empyema in nontransplant populations.[23]

Outcomes examined in the Cleveland Clinic series included eradication of infection (in subjects for whom the operative indication was empyema), lung re-expansion, and survival. Nine of 14 subjects with empyema had infection cleared, whereas the other 5 died. Interestingly, lung re-expansion and survival following decortication varied according to time from transplant. Whereas complete lung re-expansion was accomplished in 19 of 27 decortications overall (70%), it occurred in 78% of subjects undergoing decortication within 90 days of transplant and only 58% of subjects having the procedure thereafter. All 10 decortications performed within the first 41 days after transplant achieved complete lung re-expansion.[6] Survival was also associated with interval between transplantation and decortication, with subjects undergoing decortication within 90 days posttransplant having a significantly better survival

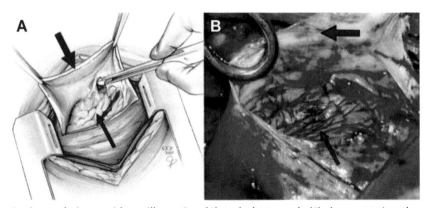

Fig. 2. Decortication technique, with an illustration (*A*) and photograph (*B*) demonstrating the cortex (*thick arrow*) being separated from the normal underlying lung (*thin arrow*). (*From* Boffa DJ, Mason DP, Su JW, et al. Decortication after lung transplantation. Ann Thorac Surg 2008;85:1040; with permission.)

than those having the operation beyond the 90 day interval (see **Fig. 1**).

Operative and postoperative complications were also studied in this series, with the main adverse perioperative outcomes being 23% operative mortality (30 days or in-house), 63% rate of renal failure, and 17% rate of new-onset atrial fibrillation. Incomplete re-expansion of the transplanted lung resulting in a residual space can be particularly problematic in the setting of a pleural space infection. These patients represent a high risk for re-infection of the residual space. In the Cleveland Clinic lung transplant series, 4 out of 15 (27%) subjects undergoing decortication for empyema were left with a residual space, of which 2 died in during hospitalization.[6] In patients with a persistent space after decortication for empyema, options include filling the space with tissue (muscle or omentum); chronic drainage; instillation of antibiotics into space and closure; or, less commonly, thoracoplasty or Clagett window. Chronic pleural drainage via a tunneled catheter or a progressively withdrawn chest tube (empyema tube) is a reasonable option for patients with a space that persists after decortication or for patients that are not candidates for surgical decortication, after the grossly infected fluid and debris have been evacuated.

This series demonstrated that decortication following lung transplantation is capable of achieving many of the traditional empyema treatment endpoints, but carries a significant cost with respect to operative mortality.

SPECIAL POPULATIONS

In addition to examining outcomes of lung transplantation overall, several series have specifically addressed special populations of subjects, including those undergoing transplantation for CF, subjects receiving living lobar transplants, and adult subjects receiving pediatric donor lungs.

Cystic Fibrosis

CF is considered a septic lung disorder, characterized by chronic recurrent respiratory infections. It has been recommended that CF patients undergoing lung transplantation receive a longer course of routine postoperative antibiotics. Many of these patients may have a pseudomonal lung infection preoperatively, and many are often colonized with multiple multidrug-resistant organisms.[24] Given the likelihood of infection or colonization at the time of operation, one of the primary concerns in CF patients undergoing lung transplantation is the development of postoperative empyema. However, CF patients have not been shown to

have a higher rate of posttransplant empyema than the general transplant population.[22] Somewhat unique, though, is that empyemas in these patients frequently demonstrate positive cultures for pseudomonas, including 100% of posttransplant empyemas in CF subjects in one study.[4]

Living Lobar Transplant Recipients

Living lobar transplantation (LLT) recipients are thought to be predisposed to pleural complications due to donor-to-recipient size mismatch, which results in greater likelihood of a postoperative airspace because a single lobe is smaller on average than a whole lung. One of the methods used to counteract this issue is to try to use donors who are taller than the recipient, with the donor lobe having a greater likelihood of filling the pleural space than a lobe from a smaller donor. Additional complicating factors in this group of patients that may predispose to pleural complications include the following: (1) the recipients essentially universally require bilateral transplantation (given the severity of disease that made LLT an option originally), (2) the recipients are more likely to have CF (76 of 84 recipients in one study), and (3) the donor lung fissure is typically divided sharply to lessen staple compression.[24]

Nevertheless, it has been shown in one study that LLT recipients have a pleural complication rate of 35%, which is not dramatically higher than the 22% to 34% rate of pleural space complications in the general transplant population. No difference in complication rate was found based on donor-to-recipient height mismatch. Within the LLT group, those with a pleural space complication had a significant longer duration of chest tube drainage (41 vs 21 days) and hospitalization (45 vs 24 days) compared with those without a pleural complication. The types of pleural complication, in descending frequency, included air leak or bronchopleural fistula (38% of pleural complications), loculated effusion (21%), pneumothorax without air leak (17%), hemothorax (13%), empyema (8%), and chylothorax (4%).[24]

Adult Recipients of Pediatric Donor Lungs

Similar to the LLT recipient group, adult recipients of pediatric donor lungs face a donor-to-recipient size mismatch that is inherently greater than that of the lung transplant recipients on the whole, resulting in the greater potential for posttransplant airspace. Keshava and colleagues[25] published the Cleveland Clinic experience with transplanting pediatric donor lungs into adult recipients. Between February 1990 and December 2007, 609 adults underwent primary lung transplantation, with 38 subjects (6.2%) receiving pediatric donor lungs. Size-matching previously included height comparison and chest radiograph comparison but has evolved to be based on the ratio of the donor predicted total lung capacity to the recipient actual total lung capacity. The feasibility of this method of size-matching was demonstrated in a previous study from Cleveland Clinic, with post-transplant survival and pulmonary function not shown to be affected by discrepancies in lung sizing.[26] In the pediatric donor series, 2 of the 38 recipients (5.3%) were considered to have received undersized donor parenchyma, while 11 (29%) received an undersized donor bronchus.

Pleural space complications were experienced in 14 of 38 subjects (37%),[25] which was slightly higher than the previously noted 22% to 34% rate of pleural complications in lung transplant recipients overall but similar to the 35% rate of pleural complications in the LLT group. Those 14 subjects required either thoracentesis (4 subjects) or tube thoracostomy (10 subjects) for pneumothorax, pleural effusion, or empyema. A total of 10 of 38 subjects (26%) in the series required reoperation, though not all for pleural space complications.[25]

SUMMARY

Despite improving outcomes overall, lung transplantation continues to result in a substantial risk of pleural space complications. Timely recognition, exclusion of associated life-threatening complications, and aggressive management are critical.

REFERENCES

1. Meyers BF, Lynch J, Trulock EP, et al. Lung transplantation: a decade of experience. Ann Surg 1999;230:362–71.
2. Van Trigt P, Davis RD, Shaeffer GS, et al. Survival benefits of heart and lung transplantation. Ann Surg 1996;223:576–84.
3. Christie JD, Edwards LB, Kucheryavaya AY, et al. The Registry of the International Society for Heart and Lung Transplantation: 29th adult lung and heart-lung transplant report—2012. J Heart Lung Transplant 2012;31:1073–86.
4. Herridge MS, de Hoyos AL, Chaparro C, et al. Pleural complications in lung transplant recipients. J Thorac Cardiovasc Surg 1995;110:22–6.
5. Ferrer J, Roldan J, Roman A, et al. Acute and chronic pleural complications in lung transplantation. J Heart Lung Transplant 2003;22:1217–25.
6. Boffa DJ, Mason DP, Su JW, et al. Decortication after lung transplantation. Ann Thorac Surg 2008;85:1039–43.
7. Marom EM, Palmer SM, Erasmus JJ, et al. Pleural effusions in lung transplant recipients: image-guided small-bore catheter drainage. Radiology 2003;228:241–5.
8. Hillerdal G. Chylothorax and pseudochylothorax. Eur Respir J 1997;10:1157–62.
9. Fremont RD, Milston AP, Light RW, et al. Chylothoraces after lung transplantation for lymphangioleiomyomatosis: review of the literature and utilization of a pleurovenous shunt. J Heart Lung Transplant 2007;26:953–5.
10. Shitrit D, Izbicki G, Fink G, et al. Late postoperative pleural effusion following lung transplantation: characteristics and clinical implications. Eur J Cardiothorac Surg 2003;23:494–6.
11. Marik PE, Pinsky M. Death by parenteral nutrition. Intensive Care Med 2003;29:867–9.
12. Boffa DJ, Sands MJ, Rice TW, et al. A critical evaluation of a percutaneous diagnostic and treatment strategy for chylothorax after thoracic surgery. Eur J Cardiothorac Surg 2008;33:435–9.
13. Siegleman SS, Sinha SB, Veith FJ. Pulmonary reimplantation response. Ann Surg 1973;177:30–6.
14. Ruggiero R, Fietsam R, Thomas GA, et al. Detection of canine allograft lung rejection by pulmonary lymphoscintigraphy. J Thorac Cardiovasc Surg 1994;108:253–8.
15. Trulock EP. Management of lung transplant rejection. Chest 1993;103:1566–76.
16. Zimmerman GS, Reithmann C, Strauss T, et al. Successful angioplasty and stent treatment of pulmonary vein stenosis after single-lung transplantation. J Heart Lung Transplant 2009;28:194–8.
17. Wahidi MM, Willner DA, Snyder LD, et al. Diagnosis and outcome of early pleural space infection following lung transplantation. Chest 2009;135:484–91.
18. Xie C, Teixeira LR, McGovern JP, et al. Systemic corticosteroids decrease the effectiveness of talc pleurodesis. Am J Respir Crit Care Med 1998;157:1441–4.
19. Teixeira LR, Wu W, Chang DS, et al. The effect of corticosteroids on pleurodesis induced by doxycycline in rabbits. Chest 2002;121:216–9.
20. Agarwal R, Aggarwal AN, Gupta D. Efficacy and safety of iodopovidone pleurodesis through tube thoracostomy. Respirology 2006;11:105–8.
21. Vakil N, Su JW, Mason DP, et al. Allograft entrapment after lung transplantation: a simple solution using a pleurocutaneous catheter. Thorac Cardiovasc Surg 2010;58:299–301.
22. Nunley DR, Grgurich WF, Keenan RJ, et al. Empyema complicating successful lung transplantation. Chest 1999;115:1312–5.
23. Striffeler H, Gugger M, Im Hof V, et al. Video-assisted thoracoscopic surgery for fibrinopurulent pleural empyema in 67 patients. Ann Thorac Surg 1998;65:319–23.

24. Backhus LM, Sievers EM, Schenkel FA, et al. Pleural space problems after living lobar transplantation. J Heart Lung Transplant 2005;24:2086–90.

25. Keshava HB, Mason DP, Murthy SC, et al. Pediatric donor lungs for adult transplant recipients: feasibility and outcomes. Thorac Cardiovasc Surg 2012;60: 275–9.

26. Mason DP, Batizy LH, Wu J, et al. Matching donor to recipient in lung transplantation: how much does size matter? J Thorac Cardiovasc Surg 2009;137:1234–40.

Reflux and Allograft Dysfunction: Is There a Connection?

 CrossMark

Brian C. Gulack, MD[a], James M. Meza, MD[a], Shu S. Lin, MD, PhD[b],
Matthew G. Hartwig, MD[c], R. Duane Davis, MD, MBA[d],*

KEYWORDS

- Lung transplantation • Gastroesophageal reflux disease • Fundoplication • Antireflux surgery
- Gastroduodenal aspiration • Allograft dysfunction • Bronchiolitis obliterans syndrome
- Chronic lung allograft dysfunction

KEY POINTS

- Patients undergoing lung transplantation have a higher rate of reflux after transplantation than before, whether caused by the surgical procedure itself or treatment-related effects (eg, immunosuppressive medications).
- Reflux following lung transplantation is associated with an increase in gastroduodenal aspiration, and this is associated with decreased lung function.
- There are limited data on the association of reflux and survival.
- Antireflux surgery is safe and the preferred method for treating documented reflux in the lung transplant population.
- Although data have demonstrated that lung function stabilizes following antireflux surgery, there is limited information with regards to survival benefit.

INTRODUCTION

Lung transplantation has seen tremendous growth since 1963 when the first lung was transplanted into a 58-year-old man suffering from squamous cell carcinoma.[1] Although the patient only survived for 18 days, it provided a new option for the treatment of patients with end-stage lung disease.[1] As of 2011, 3640 single and bilateral orthotopic lung transplantations were being performed per year.[2] Survival has steadily increased and as of 2013, median survival following transplantation was 5.6 years, up from 5.3 years in 2010.[2,3] Despite improving success, certain complications associated with lung transplantation continue to limit optimal survival. Earliest among these is primary graft dysfunction, which is defined as hypoxia, pulmonary edema, and pulmonary infiltrates that occur immediately following transplantation.[4] Although often transient, it continues to be a significant source of early mortality.[5]

BRONCHIOLITIS OBLITERANS SYNDROME

Following the acute period, most morbidity and mortality in lung transplantation is associated with either infectious complications or the development of bronchiolitis obliterans.[6] Bronchiolitis

Disclosure: The authors have nothing to disclose.
[a] Department of Surgery, Duke University Medical Center, 3443, Durham, NC 27710, USA; [b] Department of Surgery, Duke University Medical Center, 3392, Durham, NC 27710, USA; [c] Department of Surgery, Duke University Medical Center, 3863, Durham, NC 27710, USA; [d] Department of Surgery, Duke University Medical Center, 3864, Durham, NC 27710, USA
* Corresponding author.
E-mail address: duane.davis@duke.edu

Thorac Surg Clin 25 (2015) 97–105
http://dx.doi.org/10.1016/j.thorsurg.2014.09.006

obliterans is a histopathologic diagnosis consisting of fibrous scaring of the lung tissue leading to a progressive decrease in the forced expiratory volume in 1 second (FEV_1).[7] This tissue-based diagnosis is consistent with most chronic rejection. Given the difficulty of obtaining a tissue diagnosis, the term bronchiolitis obliterans syndrome (BOS) was devised to account for patients demonstrating a progressive reduction in airflow (decreasing FEV_1) following lung transplantation without another identifiable cause.[7,8] BOS is categorized by five distinct stages each defined by a percent reduction from baseline FEV_1 or forced expiratory flow between 25% and 75% of the forced vital capacity (FEF_{25-75}; **Table 1**).[7,9]

More recently, a new terminology has been developed to categorize patients with declining allograft function termed chronic lung allograft dysfunction, which includes BOS along with other less characteristic forms of persistently decreased lung function (**Fig. 1**).[10] Furthermore, restrictive allograft syndrome, a subset of chronic lung allograft dysfunction with a physiologically different presentation than BOS, has been demonstrated to have even worse survival than most patients with chronic lung allograft dysfunction.[11] These patients present with more restrictive findings on pulmonary function testing, often characterized as a decline in total lung capacity.[11]

Numerous factors have been associated with the development of BOS, including chronic rejection, repeat episodes of acute rejection, infection, and gastroesophageal reflux disease (GERD).[12-14] Hartwig and colleagues[14] demonstrated that patients with abnormal pH probe testing had increased rates of decline in their FEV_1 following lung transplantation, and that this decline was significantly worse if patients did not undergo fundoplication. Despite these data and evidence from other single institution studies, it has only been demonstrated that there is an association between reflux and allograft dysfunction, not a cause-effect relationship. This article reviews the current evidence regarding the role of reflux in allograft dysfunction (**Box 1**).

REFLUX FOLLOWING LUNG TRANSPLANTATION

For the purposes of this article, "reflux" is referred to as contents that are of a gastroduodenal nature that regurgitate up the esophagus into the pharynx. The hypothetical role of reflux in the development of BOS is because of aspiration, or the inhalation of reflux contents into the lungs. For obvious reasons, aspiration of either gastric or duodenal contents into the allograft can lead to substantial harm. Unfortunately, significant evidence has demonstrated that lung transplantation itself may increase the rate of reflux. For instance, Young and colleagues[15] demonstrated significant increases in abnormal acid contact during 24-hour pH monitoring following lung transplantation compared with before. Furthermore, studies have demonstrated reflux is increased in patients undergoing bilateral lung transplantation compared with single lung transplantation, and increased reflux is also seen in patients undergoing retransplantation as compared with primary transplantation.[16,17] Lastly, Ward and colleagues[18] and Stovold and colleagues[19] demonstrated that, compared with nontransplant recipients, post–lung transplant patients have increased levels of pepsin, a protein produced in the stomach, in bronchoalveolar lavage (BAL) fluid, although whether this is caused by the transplant or the underlying diagnosis is unclear. Together, these studies suggest that some process of the surgical procedure may increase the rate of reflux. It has been hypothesized that, because of the anatomic proximity of the vagal nerve to the surgical site, this may be caused by vagal nerve manipulation, which is known to cause issues with gastroparesis and reflux following several upper abdominal surgeries.[20-22] Alternatively, it may be secondary to the side effects of immunosuppression required for transplantation.[21]

Nonacid Reflux

Although pH monitoring is traditionally associated with the diagnosis of reflux, there is also significant

Table 1	
Classification of bronchiolitis obliterans syndrome	
BOS Classification	**Diagnostic Criteria**
BOS 0	FEV_1 >90% and FEF_{25-75} >75% of baseline
BOS 0-p	FEV_1 81%–90% and/or FEF_{25-75} ≤75% of baseline
BOS 1	FEV_1 66%–80% of baseline
BOS 2	FEV_1 51%–65% of baseline
BOS 3	FEV_1 ≤50% of baseline

Abbreviations: FEF_{25-75}, forced expiratory flow between 25% and 75% of the forced vital capacity; FEV_1, forced expiratory volume in 1 second.

Data from Estenne M, Maurer JR, Boehler A, et al. Bronchiolitis obliterans syndrome 2001: an update of the diagnostic criteria. J Heart Lung Transplant 2002;21:297–310; and Bando K, Paradis IL, Similo S, et al. Obliterative bronchiolitis after lung and heart-lung transplantation. An analysis of risk factors and management. J Thorac Cardiovasc Surg 1995;110:4–13 [discussion: 13–4].

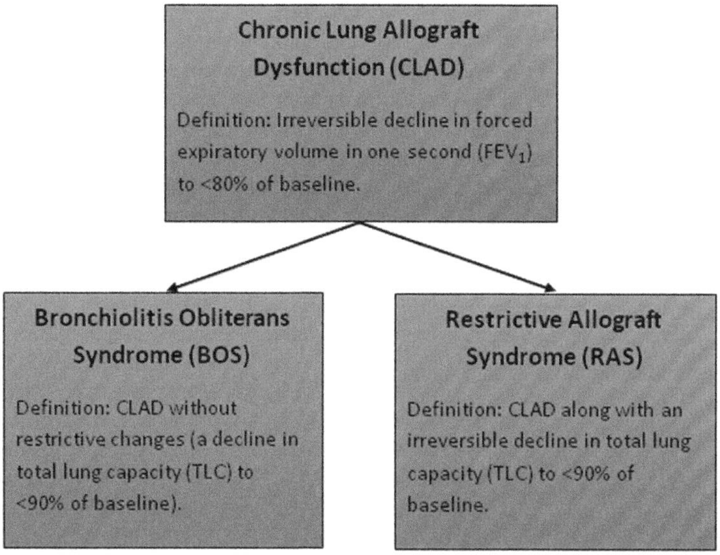

Chronic Lung Allograft
Dysfunction (CLAD)

Definition: Irreversible decline in forced
expiratory volume in one second (FEV_1)
to <80% of baseline.

Bronchiolitis Obliterans
Syndrome (BOS)

Definition: CLAD without
restrictive changes (a decline in
total lung capacity (TLC) to
<90% of baseline).

Restrictive Allograft
Syndrome (RAS)

Definition: CLAD along with an
irreversible decline in total lung
capacity (TLC) to <90% of
baseline.

Fig. 1. New classification of lung allograft dysfunction. (*Adapted from* Sato M, Waddell TK, Wagnetz U, et al. Restrictive allograft syndrome (RAS): a novel form of chronic lung allograft dysfunction. J Heart Lung Transplant 2011;30:299; with permission.)

evidence that nonacid reflux is also increased in the lung transplant population. Blondeau and colleagues[23] demonstrated that of 45 patients post–lung transplantation not on proton pump inhibitor therapy, six (13.3%) had increased nonacid reflux. Furthermore, Reder and colleagues[24] demonstrated that traditional symptoms of GERD, such as heartburn and regurgitation, had very poor sensitivity or specificity for predicting the presence of pepsin or bile in BAL in patients following lung transplantation. There is also significant evidence that when the acidity is removed from reflux, mainly through histamine blockers or proton pump inhibitors, the negative effects of reflux and aspiration are not negated. Tang and colleagues[25] performed a study on a rat lung transplant model, comparing the effects of aspiration of acidic gastric fluid, neutral gastric fluid, or saline, and found that there was no significant difference in the development of lesions consistent with bronchiolitis obliterans between rats in the neutral

pH and acidic pH groups, but there was a significant increase in both groups compared with the saline control group.

Esophageal Dysmotility

Although unclear, some evidence indicates that esophageal motility may also be associated with reflux in this patient population. Davis and colleagues[17] demonstrated in a small institutional study that of patients who had reflux diagnosed via pH monitoring, 36% also had esophageal dysmotility compared with only 6% of the patients without reflux. One hypothesis posits that the vagal nerve manipulation described previously leads to this motility issue. However, this is not entirely clear, and it may be secondary to other nontechnical reasons.

Delayed Gastric Emptying

Similar to changes in esophageal motility, there are also changes in gastric emptying following lung transplantation that are likely secondary to neuropathic issues, but once again could be secondary to a nontechnical cause, such as immunosuppression medication.[21] Berkowitz and colleagues[21] demonstrated that 9 of 38 patients developed gastroparesis following lung or heart-lung transplantation, and 44% of these patients developed BOS. The gastroparesis seen in this patient population may also be associated with the patient's pretransplant diagnosis and comorbidities, because Raviv and colleagues[26] demonstrated that around 50% of lung transplant patients have diagnostic delayed gastric emptying before transplant; however, the process of

---

Box 1
Evidence lung transplantation increases rates of reflux

- Increased rates of acid contact on pH testing in patients following transplant compared with before.
- Increased rates of reflux following bilateral lung transplantation compared with single lung transplantation.
- Increased levels of pepsin in the lungs of transplant patients compared with nontransplant patients.

transplantation does increase this number to 74% at 3 months. Nevertheless, a significant portion of the newly diagnosed population returns to normal with time.[26]

Mucociliary Clearance

In addition to increased rates of reflux, lung transplantation has also been associated with decreased rates of mucociliary clearance. This may compound the negative effect of gastroduodenal aspiration on lung transplant recipients compared with the normal population, because once contents are aspirated, they are less likely to be cleared.[21,27] Similar to other physiologic changes discussed previously, impaired mucociliary clearance in lung transplant recipients may be secondary to allograft denervation or to side effects of antirejection medications.[28,29]

Risk Factors Associated with Increased Reflux

Multiple patient-related factors have also been implicated in reflux disease in addition to the operative procedures (bilateral vs single lung transplantation, retransplantation vs primary transplantation) listed previously. Perhaps most importantly, certain diagnoses have been found to be associated with much higher rates of reflux following lung transplantation (**Box 2**). Patients with connective tissue disorders have been found to have very high rates of acid reflux and esophageal dysmotility before and after transplantation.[30] Furthermore, patients with cystic fibrosis, the third most common indication for lung transplantation, also have a much higher rate of acid reflux than patients with other diagnoses.[3,31] Mendez and colleagues[31] demonstrated that patients with a diagnosis of cystic fibrosis have rates of acid reflux around 90% posttransplant, whereas the same is true in only 54% of patients with other diagnoses.

PATHOPHYSIOLOGY OF REFLUX AND ALLOGRAFT DYSFUNCTION

Although there is significant evidence that the incidence of reflux is increased in the lung transplant population, it is unclear what the exact mechanism is that may lead to allograft dysfunction. Next, three different proposed hypotheses of how gastroduodenal aspiration may lead to allograft

---

> **Box 2**
> **Diagnoses associated with increased rates of reflux**
>
> • Cystic fibrosis
> • Connective tissue disorders

---

injury are reviewed (**Fig. 2**). One hypothesis posits that the reflux particulates themselves may cause a chemical injury on aspiration.[32] A second hypothesis suggests that bile acid aspiration leads to an impairment in the innate immune system in the lung tissue. D'Ovidio and colleagues[33] found that patients with high levels of bile acids on BAL also had significantly lower levels of surfactant molecules, surfactant protein A and surfactant protein D, phosphatidylglycerol, and dipalmitoylphosphatidylcholine, and significantly higher levels of sphingomyelin. Surfactant protein D and surfactant protein D are known to be involved in the opsonization of organisms and are also involved in the regulation of cytokines involved in the immune response.[33] The phospholipids described previously are involved in creating a physical barrier for pulmonary tissue, which when disrupted, can increase the incidence of pulmonary damage from other factors.[33]

A third hypothesis contends that the contents of the aspirate promote an inflammatory milieu, which in turn leads to allograft rejection and dysfunction by stimulating nonalloimmune injury. Li and colleagues[34] demonstrated that the levels of interleukin-1α, tumor necrosis factor-α, and transforming growth factor-$\beta1$ were significantly elevated in the BAL of a rat lung transplant model undergoing gastric fluid aspiration compared with control subjects. Furthermore, levels of interleukin-1α, interleukin-4, and granulocyte-macrophage colony–stimulating factor were significantly elevated in the serum of these rat models.[34] This cytokine cascade of known proinflammatory cytokines caused by chronic gastric fluid aspiration may lead to the eventual development of fibrosis and BOS. Meltzer and colleagues[35] later performed this study in a swine model and found that repeat gastric aspiration led to shedding of alloantigens. This highlights a possible mechanism for how a nonspecific inflammatory response can lead to an increase in specific alloresponse against the allograft. Furthermore, at least one model demonstrated the development of bronchiolitis obliterans following repeated gastric fluid aspiration.

Although multiple hypotheses exist with regards to the exact pathophysiology of lung injury from gastroduodenal aspiration, it is likely not explainable by a single mechanism, but more likely a combination of mechanisms. Reflux likely causes direct injury independently, and by weakening the allograft's innate immune system, thereby decreasing its ability to fight off infection. Furthermore, the reflux likely causes cellular activation and cytokine production, thus causing cellular damage through inflammatory mediators.

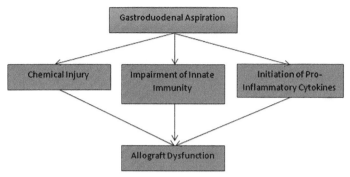

Fig. 2. Diagram representing the three hypothesized pathways by which gastroduodenal aspiration may lead to allograft dysfunction.

OUTCOMES RELATED TO REFLUX

Although limited by small sample sizes, some studies have found correlations between reflux and specific outcomes, including acute rejection and BOS (**Box 3**).[36,37]

Acute Rejection

A few studies have been performed to determine the association of reflux and acute rejection. Shah and colleagues[36] found that GERD as defined as a DeMeester score greater than 14.7 was significantly associated with single and multiple (two or more) acute rejection episodes. Furthermore, Fisichella and colleagues,[38] in a prospective single institution study, found that aspiration, defined as pepsin present in BAL, was correlated with a significantly higher acute rejection rate. Lastly, Stovold and colleagues[19] measured pepsin levels on BAL and found that they were significantly higher in patients with acute rejection.

Bronchiolitis Obliterans Syndrome

In addition to acute rejection, there is evidence of an association of BOS with reflux and aspiration. The multitude of these studies are retrospective reviews of a lung transplant population, and unfortunately there was significant variation in the definition of GERD, some using esophagogastroduodenoscopy, whereas others based the diagnosis on pH monitoring. Most found some correlation with reflux and BOS, but not necessarily with the tissue diagnosis of bronchiolitis obliterans.[37,39] A few studies have also been performed in a prospective manner, once again finding a similar correlation between reflux and BOS.[14,19,33,38]

Survival

Although there is substantial evidence of a correlation between gastroduodenal aspiration and BOS, there is a less clear effect on overall survival. This is likely secondary to studies limited by small sample size. However, one retrospective study was able to demonstrate this effect. Murthy and colleagues[40] performed a retrospective study at their institution of 215 patients, and found that patients with GERD by preoperative pH testing had a significantly worse survival compared with those with a negative preoperative pH test. Although significant, further investigation is necessary to document a clear correlation between gastroduodenal aspiration and survival. Key takeaways are noted in **Box 4**.

PREVENTION AND TREATMENT OF GASTROESOPHAGEAL REFLUX DISEASE

Despite limited evidence that reflux leading to gastroduodenal aspiration is associated with

---

Box 3
Reflux following lung transplantation has been associated with various outcomes

- Acute rejection
- Decreased FEV_1
- Bronchiolitis obliterans syndrome
- Survival

Box 4
Take-home points

- Multiple studies have found associations between reflux and BOS.
- Fewer studies have been able to document a correlation with survival.
- No study to date has demonstrated causality.

decreased survival, there is substantial support for the treatment of reflux following lung transplantation. This can include medical and surgical therapies (**Fig. 3**).

Medical Therapy

The basis for medical therapy to treat reflux is traditionally oriented around decreasing the acidity of gastric contents, most commonly with histamine blockers or proton pump inhibitors.[41,42] Although these are very effective at reducing symptomatology, there is growing evidence that nonacid components of reflux also lead to significant damage and augment GERD-associated pulmonary injury.[43] That being said, a large proportion of transplant patients begin antacid therapy postoperatively. Whether this provides any benefit is unknown, but there is concern that it may mask symptoms of reflux and lead to silent aspiration, thereby increasing the risk of BOS and possibly decreasing survival.[23] Furthermore, there is some evidence that antacid therapy may lead to bacterial overgrowth of the gastrointestinal tract, which may further increase the injury to the allograft associated with aspiration.[44]

In addition to antacids, azithromycin has also been used in the treatment of BOS.[45] Azithromycin, an antibiotic used for a variety of bacterial infections, has been demonstrated to have anti-inflammatory and prokinetic properties.[46,47] Leading to an increase in esophageal and gastric motility, azithromycin has been demonstrated to be beneficial in the treatment of BOS, although

the exact mechanism responsible for this is unclear.[47,48]

Antireflux Surgery

Antacid therapy to neutralize gastric contents likely only blunts the effect of gastroduodenal aspiration on allograft function, and may actually lead to an increase in silent aspiration of nonacid reflux.[25] Consequently, many transplant physicians recommend the use of antireflux surgery, specifically fundoplication, in patients diagnosed with reflux to prevent acidic and nonacidic components of reflux from being aspirated.[14]

Although initially there were concerns regarding the safety of antireflux surgery in this population, many studies have demonstrated very low associated morbidity and mortality.[22,30,49,50] Furthermore, antireflux surgery has been shown to lead to a significant reduction in immune modulators associated with the development of BOS, and preservation in overall lung function.[14,22,51,52] The benefit of fundoplication is likely maximized if performed earlier rather than later following transplant, to limit the amount of time gastroduodenal aspiration has to affect the allograft.[14] Despite this anecdotal evidence, only one study has yet to demonstrate a survival benefit in patients who undergo antireflux surgery. Cantu and colleagues[53] demonstrated that patients with a diagnosis of GERD who undergo early fundoplication (within 90 days) had a significantly increased survival at 1 year than patients with a later fundoplication or no fundoplication.

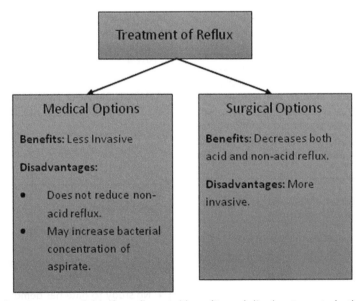

Fig. 3. Overview of treatments available for reflux, and benefits and disadvantages to both.

SUMMARY

The association between reflux and allograft function has seen significant debate in the literature. Unfortunately, because of the small sample sizes inherent to this patient population, few studies have definitively demonstrated a survival effect related to reflux, or a benefit from its prevention. As stated by Fisichella and colleagues,[54] the current literature "supports only a strong association between GERD [gastroesophageal reflux disease] and BOS, but not causality." Further investigation is needed before a definitive answer can be determined. However, what can be gleaned from the current status of literature on this topic is that there is likely a relationship between reflux and gastroduodenal aspiration; that this aspiration leads to significant allograft dysfunction, which likely affects survival; and that there may be benefit from surgical, but not necessarily medical, treatment of reflux.

REFERENCES

1. Hardy JD, Webb WR, Dalton ML Jr, et al. Lung homotransplantation in man. JAMA 1963;186:1065–74.
2. Yusen RD, Christie JD, Edwards LB, et al. The registry of the International Society for Heart and Lung Transplantation: thirtieth adult lung and heart-lung transplant report–2013; focus theme: age. J Heart Lung Transplant 2013;32:965–78.
3. Christie JD, Edwards LB, Kucheryavaya AY, et al. The registry of the International Society for Heart and Lung Transplantation: twenty-seventh official adult lung and heart-lung transplant report–2010. J Heart Lung Transplant 2010;29:1104–18.
4. Christie JD, Bavaria JE, Palevsky HI, et al. Primary graft failure following lung transplantation. Chest 1998;114:51–60.
5. Christie JD, Sager JS, Kimmel SE, et al. Impact of primary graft failure on outcomes following lung transplantation. Chest 2005;127:161–5.
6. Meyers BF, de la Morena M, Sweet SC, et al. Primary graft dysfunction and other selected complications of lung transplantation: a single-center experience of 983 patients. J Thorac Cardiovasc Surg 2005; 129:1421–9.
7. Estenne M, Maurer JR, Boehler A, et al. Bronchiolitis obliterans syndrome 2001: an update of the diagnostic criteria. J Heart Lung Transplant 2002;21: 297–310.
8. Cooper JD, Billingham M, Egan T, et al. A working formulation for the standardization of nomenclature and for clinical staging of chronic dysfunction in lung allografts. International Society for Heart and Lung Transplantation. J Heart Lung Transplant 1993;12:713–6.
9. Bando K, Paradis IL, Similo S, et al. Obliterative bronchiolitis after lung and heart-lung transplantation. An analysis of risk factors and management. J Thorac Cardiovasc Surg 1995;110:4–13 [discussion: 13–4].
10. Todd JL, Jain R, Pavlisko EN, et al. Impact of forced vital capacity loss on survival after the onset of chronic lung allograft dysfunction. Am J Respir Crit Care Med 2014;189:159–66.
11. Sato M, Waddell TK, Wagnetz U, et al. Restrictive allograft syndrome (RAS): a novel form of chronic lung allograft dysfunction. J Heart Lung Transplant 2011;30:735–42.
12. Chalermskulrat W, Neuringer IP, Schmitz JL, et al. Human leukocyte antigen mismatches predispose to the severity of bronchiolitis obliterans syndrome after lung transplantation. Chest 2003; 123:1825–31.
13. Keller CA, Cagle PT, Brown RW, et al. Bronchiolitis obliterans in recipients of single, double, and heart-lung transplantation. Chest 1995;107:973–80.
14. Hartwig MG, Anderson DJ, Onaitis MW, et al. Fundoplication after lung transplantation prevents the allograft dysfunction associated with reflux. Ann Thorac Surg 2011;92:462–8 [discussion: 468–9].
15. Young LR, Hadjiliadis D, Davis RD, et al. Lung transplantation exacerbates gastroesophageal reflux disease. Chest 2003;124:1689–93.
16. Fisichella PM, Davis CS, Shankaran V, et al. The prevalence and extent of gastroesophageal reflux disease correlates to the type of lung transplantation. Surg Laparosc Endosc Percutan Tech 2012; 22:46–51.
17. Davis CS, Shankaran V, Kovacs EJ, et al. Gastroesophageal reflux disease after lung transplantation: pathophysiology and implications for treatment. Surgery 2010;148:737–44 [discussion: 744–5].
18. Ward C, Forrest IA, Brownlee IA, et al. Pepsin like activity in bronchoalveolar lavage fluid is suggestive of gastric aspiration in lung allografts. Thorax 2005; 60:872–4.
19. Stovold R, Forrest IA, Corris PA, et al. Pepsin, a biomarker of gastric aspiration in lung allografts: a putative association with rejection. Am J Respir Crit Care Med 2007;175:1298–303.
20. Shafi MA, Pasricha PJ. Post-surgical and obstructive gastroparesis. Curr Gastroenterol Rep 2007;9: 280–5.
21. Berkowitz N, Schulman LL, McGregor C, et al. Gastroparesis after lung transplantation. Potential role in postoperative respiratory complications. Chest 1995;108:1602–7.
22. Robertson AG, Krishnan A, Ward C, et al. Anti-reflux surgery in lung transplant recipients: outcomes and effects on quality of life. Eur Respir J 2012;39:691–7.
23. Blondeau K, Mertens V, Vanaudenaerde BA, et al. Gastro-oesophageal reflux and gastric aspiration in

lung transplant patients with or without chronic rejection. Eur Respir J 2008;31:707–13.

24. Reder NP, Davis CS, Kovacs EJ, et al. The diagnostic value of gastroesophageal reflux disease (GERD) symptoms and detection of pepsin and bile acids in bronchoalveolar lavage fluid and exhaled breath condensate for identifying lung transplantation patients with GERD-induced aspiration. Surg Endosc 2014;28(6):1794–800.

25. Tang T, Chang JC, Xie A, et al. Aspiration of gastric fluid in pulmonary allografts: effect of pH. J Surg Res 2013;181:e31–8.

26. Raviv Y, D'Ovidio F, Pierre A, et al. Prevalence of gastroparesis before and after lung transplantation and its association with lung allograft outcomes. Clin Transplant 2012;26:133–42.

27. D'Ovidio F, Mura M, Tsang M, et al. Bile acid aspiration and the development of bronchiolitis obliterans after lung transplantation. J Thorac Cardiovasc Surg 2005;129:1144–52.

28. Pazetti R, Pego-Fernandes PM, Jatene FB. Adverse effects of immunosuppressant drugs upon airway epithelial cell and mucociliary clearance: implications for lung transplant recipients. Drugs 2013;73:1157–69.

29. Bhashyam AR, Mogayzel PJ Jr, Cleary JC, et al. Vagal control of mucociliary clearance in murine lungs: a study in a chronic preparation. Auton Neurosci 2010;154:74–8.

30. Gasper WJ, Sweet MP, Golden JA, et al. Lung transplantation in patients with connective tissue disorders and esophageal dysmotility. Dis Esophagus 2008;21:650–5.

31. Mendez BM, Davis CS, Weber C, et al. Gastroesophageal reflux disease in lung transplant patients with cystic fibrosis. Am J Surg 2012;204:e21–6.

32. Neujahr DC, Uppal K, Force SD, et al. Bile acid aspiration associated with lung chemical profile linked to other biomarkers of injury after lung transplantation. Am J Transplant 2014;14:841–8.

33. D'Ovidio F, Mura M, Ridsdale R, et al. The effect of reflux and bile acid aspiration on the lung allograft and its surfactant and innate immunity molecules Sp-A and Sp-D. Am J Transplant 2006;6:1930–8.

34. Li B, Hartwig MG, Appel JZ, et al. Chronic aspiration of gastric fluid induces the development of obliterative bronchiolitis in rat lung transplants. Am J Transplant 2008;8:1614–21.

35. Meltzer AJ, Weiss MJ, Veillette GR, et al. Repetitive gastric aspiration leads to augmented indirect allorecognition after lung transplantation in miniature swine. Transplantation 2008;86:1824–9.

36. Shah N, Force SD, Mitchell PO, et al. Gastroesophageal reflux disease is associated with an increased rate of acute rejection in lung transplant allografts. Transplant Proc 2010;42:2702–6.

37. Molina EJ, Short S, Monteiro G, et al. Symptomatic gastroesophageal reflux disease after lung transplantation. Gen Thorac Cardiovasc Surg 2009;57:647–53.

38. Fisichella PM, Davis CS, Lundberg PW, et al. The protective role of laparoscopic antireflux surgery against aspiration of pepsin after lung transplantation. Surgery 2011;150:598–606.

39. Hadjiliadis D, Duane Davis R, Steele MP, et al. Gastroesophageal reflux disease in lung transplant recipients. Clin Transplant 2003;17:363–8.

40. Murthy SC, Nowicki ER, Mason DP, et al. Preoperative Gastroesophageal Reflux Impacts Early Outcomes after Lung Transplantation. The Journal of Heart and Lung Transplantation 2009;28(2):s214.

41. Sabesin SM, Berlin RG, Humphries TJ, et al. Famotidine relieves symptoms of gastroesophageal reflux disease and heals erosions and ulcerations. Results of a multicenter, placebo-controlled, dose-ranging study. USA Merck Gastroesophageal Reflux Disease Study Group. Arch Intern Med 1991;151:2394–400.

42. Robinson M. Review article: the pharmacodynamics and pharmacokinetics of proton pump inhibitors: overview and clinical implications. Aliment Pharmacol Ther 2004;20(Suppl 6):1–10.

43. Fahim A, Crooks M, Hart SP. Gastroesophageal reflux and idiopathic pulmonary fibrosis: a review. Pulm Med 2011;2011:634613.

44. Theisen J, Nehra D, Citron D, et al. Suppression of gastric acid secretion in patients with gastroesophageal reflux disease results in gastric bacterial overgrowth and deconjugation of bile acids. J Gastrointest Surg 2000;4:50–4.

45. Gerhardt SG, McDyer JF, Girgis RE, et al. Maintenance azithromycin therapy for bronchiolitis obliterans syndrome: results of a pilot study. Am J Respir Crit Care Med 2003;168:121–5.

46. Fisichella PM, Jalilvand A. The role of impaired esophageal and gastric motility in end-stage lung diseases and after lung transplantation. J Surg Res 2014;186:201–6.

47. Vos R, Vanaudenaerde BM, Verleden SE, et al. Anti-inflammatory and immunomodulatory properties of azithromycin involved in treatment and prevention of chronic lung allograft rejection. Transplantation 2012;94:101–9.

48. Vos R, Vanaudenaerde BM, Verleden SE, et al. A randomised controlled trial of azithromycin to prevent chronic rejection after lung transplantation. Eur Respir J 2011;37:164–72.

49. Abbassi-Ghadi N, Kumar S, Cheung B, et al. Anti-reflux surgery for lung transplant recipients in the presence of impedance-detected duodenogastroesophageal reflux and bronchiolitis obliterans syndrome: a study of efficacy and safety. J Heart Lung Transplant 2013;32:588–95.

50. Fisichella PM, Davis CS, Gagermeier J, et al. Laparoscopic antireflux surgery for gastroesophageal reflux disease after lung transplantation. J Surg Res 2011;170:e279–86.
51. Fisichella PM, Davis CS, Lowery E, et al. Pulmonary immune changes early after laparoscopic antireflux surgery in lung transplant patients with gastroesophageal reflux disease. J Surg Res 2012;177:e65–73.
52. Neujahr DC, Mohammed A, Ulukpo O, et al. Surgical correction of gastroesophageal reflux in lung transplant patients is associated with decreased effector CD8 Cells in lung lavages: a case series. Chest 2010;138:937–43.
53. Cantu E III, Appel JZ III, Hartwig MG, et al. J. Maxwell Chamberlain memorial paper. Early fundoplication prevents chronic allograft dysfunction in patients with gastroesophageal reflux disease. Ann Thorac Surg 2004;78:1142–51 [discussion: 1142–51].
54. Fisichella PM, Davis CS, Kovacs EJ. A review of the role of gerd-induced aspiration after lung transplantation. Surg Endosc 2012;26:1201–4.

Artificial Lungs
Are We There yet?

Martin Strueber, MD

KEYWORDS

• Lung • Circulatory support • Heart failure • Oxygenation

KEY POINTS

- New oxygenator technologies widened the application of extracorporeal life support significantly in the last decade.
- Currently the use is still limited within intensive care units.
- Compared to ventricular assist devices for heart failure, lung replacement technology is lagging behind, not allowing discharge on device.
- Challenges to achieve a true artificial lung for long term use are discussed in this article.

INTRODUCTION

The last decade has seen a change in the clinical use of circulatory support for heart failure. Technical improvements have made it possible to move from a short-term bridge to transplantation to use in chronic therapy.[1] Although it is not a perfect solution, with a high incidence of adverse events, it allows patients to live on chronic support at home for several years. If this scale of expectations is applied to pulmonary support, the answer to the question "Are we there yet?" is "No."

This article describes the history of pulmonary support, the technical changes, and the clinical indications and discusses the common adverse events. In addition, about it discusses what needs to be improved for pulmonary support to be used as a long-term lung assist device.

HISTORY: DEVELOPMENT OF OXYGENATORS

The development of so-called artificial lungs for clinical use was linked very early with the development of a heart-lung machine for heart

surgery. An oxygenator for gas exchange was the limiting factor in the development of these machines.

The task was to design a reliable machine to oxygenate and decarboxylate blood. It was preferable for it to be a disposable item to avoid the expensive and time-consuming cleaning and sterilizing processes.

Decarboxylation occurs easily by diffusion, but oxygenation is a difficult task because it[2] requires contact of oxygen with thin layers of blood. For about a century the technical solutions were based on direct contact of oxygen with blood. In 1882 the first experimental so-called bubble oxygenator was developed along with a two-dimensional film oxygenator.[3] After decades of research the first clinical applications using a large stationary screen oxygenator by Gibbon[4,5] were done in 1953, in which a stable film of blood was exposed to a flow of oxygen. This development was a major change of paradigms in cardiac surgery.[6] After these initial applications the bubble oxygenator emerged as the main choice of design, which was a key step in the development of open heart surgery. It allowed heart surgery programs to be

Disclosure: The author has nothing to disclose.
Heart and Lung Transplantation, Heart Failure Surgery and MCS Richard DeVos Heart&Lung Transplant Program Spectrum Health Hospitals, 330 Barclay Avenue NE, Grand Rapids, MI 49503, USA
E-mail address: strm@med.uni-leipzig.de

Thorac Surg Clin 25 (2015) 107–113
http://dx.doi.org/10.1016/j.thorsurg.2014.09.009
1547-4127/15/$ – see front matter © 2015 Elsevier Inc. All rights reserved.

thoracic.theclinics.com

established worldwide and was still in use in the 1980s.

It became clear that a limiting factor in the use of extracorporeal gas exchange was blood trauma.[7] Unlike the experience with cross-circulation from other humans, mechanical blood trauma became (and still is) an issue: hemolysis was the key factor in limiting the time of use. Additional trauma to blood constituents, like damage to the coagulation system and the induction of an inflammatory response, limited the time of use to several hours and caused severe bleeding events.[8]

A different idea was that bubbles are harmful to the blood and a system similar to a dialysis membrane, resembling the natural lung, carrying oxygen to the blood and removing CO_2 would be better.[9]

When the first membrane oxygenators were developed, which improved biocompatibility by avoiding direct air/blood contact and making longer-term use feasible, the application for lung failure was seen immediately and the extracorporeal membrane oxygenation (ECMO) was introduced into clinical practice. However, after some encouraging reports, a clinical trial in 1975 to 1977 revealed disappointing results.[10] Therefore the use of ECMO remained controversial.

In the 1980s new designs emerged: the microporous hollow fiber membrane and the dense silicone membranes.

When these oxygenators were used for heart surgery the area of the membranes and the transmembranous pressure gradient were substantial, so pumps in the heart-lung machines had to overcome the pressure gradient not only from venous return to arterial outflows but also through oxygenator membranes. In addition, the large foreign surface areas triggered an inflammatory response. Stability of the membranes was also a problem: significant losses of plasma.

Despite these limitations, membrane oxygenators were the technical development that allowed the successful introduction of ECMO for lung failure.[11]

Closed circuits were designed from components of the heart-lung machine, including a pump and membrane oxygenators.[12] Because pressure gradients across these machines were critical, some strategies were designed to allow long-term use.

The pressure gradient consists of the delta of arterial and venous blood pressure in addition to the pressure gradient induced by the circuit tubing, and especially the oxygenator. By using this device for a venovenous approach, the pressure gradient from venous to arterial system was therefore eliminated from the equation.

This simple strategy is still one of the main reasons to prefer a venovenous rather than a venoarterial approach. Second, by using 2 oxygenators in parallel, the overall pressure gradient was significantly reduced. The trade-off is the increase in foreign surface area. It was used in many centers[13] because the gain in hemocompatibility was high, especially when greater blood flows were required. In addition, the reliability of oxygenators for long-term use was limited in the 1980s by possible plasma leaks and blood coagulation, so having a second oxygenator in a parallel circle added safety to the system and allowed easy membrane exchange.

With current technology this is no longer required (discussed later).

Silicone membranes seemed to be more stable for long-term use, but their high pressure gradient turned out to be limiting.

This new technology allowed use in patients with acute lung injury and adult respiratory distress syndrome. In addition, it was also used for infants in acute lung[14] failure and in patients after cardiotomy failure.

The predominant indication was respiratory failure despite mechanical ventilation and the aim was to bridge to recovery.

At the same time (1980s) lung transplantation emerged as a clinical reality. However, the experience was limited and the preservation of lungs was still an issue. At that time numerous studies on lung preservation were initiated indicating the need for improvement. The clinical problem was a high incidence of primary graft failure, so even in the early stages ECMO was immediately introduced into lung transplant programs to either bridge to recovery or to early retransplantation.[15]

Most of the time in primary graft failure the ECMO was used in a venoarterial mode to reduce pulmonary blood flow (with the limitations discussed earlier). Despite reports of success in limited series the overall outcome was so poor that some centers decided not to use this technology.

The next step in the evolution was the introduction of new pump technologies derived from cardiac support and improvements of the tubing surfaces.

However, more important was the introduction of a new membrane type for oxygenators: the polymethylpentene membranes. These membranes became the oxygenators of choice for ECMO therapy around the world. The advantages were the absence of plasma leakage, the 5-fold to 10-fold reduction in pressure (only 11–15 mm Hg at 2.5 L of blood flow), the ease of use, and the safety when operated with a modern centrifugal pump.

These advantages were revolutionary and suggested new applications (**Figs. 1** and **2**).[16]

At first it was introduced as a pumpless lung assist device driven by the arterial pressure of the patient. Only a (percutaneous) cannulation in the groin was required to connect the system to the venous and arterial systems. It proved to be effective to eliminate CO_2 and added some oxygenation. Thereby ventilator-induced trauma could be reduced by removing CO_2 with the new system.[17]

When we used this method as a bridge to transplantation in young recipients with cystic fibrosis, the recipients were mechanically ventilated and the cutoff point for the system was an arterial CO_2 of 100 mm Hg. We learned that such a state could rapidly be reversed by this system.[18] In addition, so-called septic states with decreased vascular resistance could be reversed by normalizing the CO_2 levels. Thereby most such patients could successfully be transplanted.

The industry moved forward in making this approach usable outside the cardiothoracic units with the development of transcutaneous cannulae and the introduction of this technology to intensivists treating patients with acute lung injury. The aim was to reduce ventilator-induced trauma of the lung by taking away the burden of gas exchange.[19]

The next step for us was the combination of the modern centrifugal blood pumps with the new oxygenators, which led to the development of miniature ECMO circuits for venovenous or venoarterial application. This step seemed necessary to increase the efficacy of oxygenation and create the least invasive machine for circulatory support. Bulky machines with backup circuits were replaced by simple pump/oxygenator combinations.[20] These ideas were appreciated by the

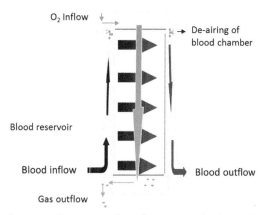

O₂ Inflow

De-airing of blood chamber

Blood reservoir

Blood inflow

Blood outflow

Gas outflow

Fig. 2. Configuration of gas flow perpendicular to the blood flow.

industry, and an integrated pump/oxygenator unit in 1 small housing became available. This miniaturization process facilitated the use of these devices for transport of patients. Extracorporeal life support centers were able to start therapy at other hospitals and transport patients into their specialized units.[21] Because of the safety of these new ECMO devices, around-the-clock monitoring by a dedicated perfusionist was no longer required, contributing to the cost-effectiveness of the procedure.

We developed an alternative approach together with the Toronto lung transplant group. In primary pulmonary hypertension a unique pathophysiology exists regarding the cardiac adaptation to the disease. In short, a severe hypertrophy of the right heart to overcome the pulmonary vascular resistance is combined with a volume-depleted left heart caused by reduced cardiac outputs. Right heart failure is usually fast and severe before transplantation, because progress in modern drug therapy has led to very advanced stages of disease when transplant is considered. The use of venoarterial ECMO may relieve the symptoms of right heart failure but further reduces the blood flow to the left ventricle. After transplantation, the full blood flow may lead to left heart failure, which may be confused with primary graft dysfunction. An alternative for such cases is to use the pulmonary artery to left atrium shunt (PA/LA) artificial lung as bridge to transplantation. Driven by the high pressures of the pulmonary artery, an extracorporeal circuit with a pumpless oxygenator can be used to overcome the symptoms. After cannulation of the pulmonary artery and the left atrium, the extracorporeal blood flow bypasses the lung and, after passing through a Polymethylpentene membrane, oxygenator, enters the left atrium. Although blood flow may range from about 1.5 to 2 L/min, it is sufficient to stabilize the circulation.

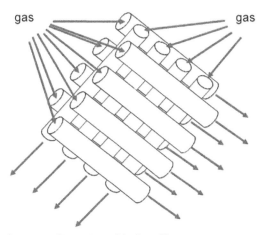

gas   gas

Fig. 1. Configuration of hollow fibers.

Bridging patients for several weeks in a nonintubated state to successful lung transplantation was reported from several centers. The connection of an additional extracorporeal circuit leads to higher blood flow to the left atrium, thereby inducing an adaptation of the left heart to volume load before transplantation.

As a further contribution, technical advances in cannulation technology allow safe percutaneous implantation techniques. This development has expanded ECMO use from the realms of cardiac and vascular surgery into intensive care units as well as interventional cardiology. Specialized cannulae designed to allow venovenous ECMO with a single double-lumen catheter have improved the efficacy of this approach.

Use of this technology for respiratory failure outside transplantation gained widespread interest and acceptance during the influenza A (H1N1) pandemic in 2009.[22]

The understanding of evolution in technology and its application over the last decade explains why there still is heterogeneity in its application in different centers in the world.

CANNULATION AND TECHNICAL ASPECTS

In emergency situations caused by circulatory or acute respiratory failure quick and easy access for ECMO can be achieved by transcutaneous femoral arterial and venous cannulation. Visualization by angiography or sonography may be necessary in some cases for safety and speed. For arterial cannulation the flow to the distal limb needs to be respected. If only partial flow is required a small cannula may help, but in general a distal perfusion catheter is recommended. Control of distal limb perfusion is mandatory after such procedures.

General anesthesia is avoidable in such cases and to cannulate with local anesthesia may be beneficial to avoid mechanical ventilation or circulatory instability. If venoarterial ECMO is used in patients to compensate for hypoxia, femoral cannulation may lead to severe hypoxia of the heart and the brain. Although the lower part of the body is oxygenated by ECMO and retrograde blood flow into the aorta, the upper part of the body may receive deoxygenated blood ejected from the heart into the ascending aorta. Therefore, it is mandatory to monitor proper oxygenation of the upper part of the body. Blood drawn from an arterial line of the right arm, or oxygen saturation measured noninvasively at the right arm or the skull, are used to ensure adequate conditions, especially in sedated patients.

If venoarterial ECMO is considered in nonemergency situations, cannulation of the right subclavian artery may be an option of choice. The advantages are a secure oxygen delivery to the brain and into the aortic root. In addition, for longer-term use and in awake patients, it may be beneficial to avoid arterial groin cannulation to allow for mobilization. Direct cannulation may be cumbersome for the small size of the artery. An end-to-side anastomosis of a short 6-mm to 8-mm vascular graft that is connected to the arterial cannula of the ECMO is preferred by some surgeons. Care must be taken not to cause a hyperperfusion of the right arm by such a procedure.

For venovenous cannulation, 2 options exist. One is the classic placement of the inflow cannula through the femoral vein to the right atrium and the outflow cannula through the jugular vein to the superior vena cava or the upper right atrium. Proper visualization is advisable by echocardiography or angiography. The outflow cannula must be of larger size for effective draining (21–28 Fr). A key factor is to avoid suction events and bad draining for efficacy of the extracorporeal circuit and avoidance of blood trauma. The inflow cannula can be substantially smaller (15–18 Fr). Efficacy of the ECMO is reduced when a substantial amount of blood flow is not drained into the ECMO and bypasses the circuit, which limits the ability to oxygenate the blood.

A newer option is to use double-lumen cannula through the right jugular vein or subclavian vein. Such cannulae are especially designed in a way that the outflow directly flows into the right ventricle and the inflow drains all venous blood returning from the body. This technique was successfully used in acute respiratory distress syndrome and may be of advantage in extubated patients, because it avoids any groin cannulation. However, proper placement and fixation of these large cannulae is the key to adequate support: at the time of placement, echocardiography is required to identify the correct location. Translocation, mostly during mobilization and movements of the patient, may compromise the function, so vigorous fixation may be required.

INDICATIONS IN LUNG TRANSPLANTATION

Before ECMO is chosen for any indication, clinicians should consider the underlying disorder and the main objective of the intervention. Is it CO_2 removal, oxygenation deficit, or circulatory failure caused by left or right heart or biventricular failure? Or is it a combination?

The next question concerns the intended time of use. Is it a bridge to recovery, a bridge to transplantation, or just a bridge to decision making? How long might this take?

The third question is about the overall status of the patient. Is there clear information about potential secondary organ failure by hypoxia or circulatory failure? Brain and kidney injury in particular may be the targets of a first assessment. If this is unclear, is a bridge to decision making indicated?

In emergencies, when there is no time for careful assessment, venoarterial ECMO is used by some centers as a first-line treatment of stabilization to allow time for further decision making (discussed earlier). In all other situations, the algorithm of decision making described earlier should apply.

If venoarterial ECMO is chosen, the time horizon of treatment is usually in the range of 1 to 2 weeks. After that, complications associated with blood trauma should be expected. In addition, problems of oxygen delivery to the heart and the brain may occur, which is when femorofemoral cannulation is used and subclavian cannulation should be considered.

In lung transplantation there are 2 major indications for ECMO: respiratory failure and right heart failure. ECMO may be used as bridge to transplantation, during the transplant procedure, or after the transplant, especially in severe primary graft dysfunction.

The main way to bridge patients deteriorating on the waiting list for transplantation is still mechanical ventilation. The success of such intervention depends on the rapid availability of a donor lung. Immobilization because of invasive ventilation leads to rapid decrease in both peripheral and chest musculature. The time to wean patients after lung transplantation is therefore a function of the time on ventilator before transplantation.

This method has been the classic way to use ECMO when patients deteriorate even while being mechanically ventilated. This approach became highly questionable because it involves selecting the patients with the highest risk for transplant.[23] Therefore, a new approach emerged that used ECMO not in addition but as an alternative to mechanical ventilation.

With current technology it seems beneficial not to intubate patients but to use ECMO in awake and ambulatory patients to maintain muscular function and oral feeding and to reduce infections.[24]

As described earlier, the combination of the artificial lung or interventional lung assist (ILA) led to a superior new generation of ECMO circuits outperforming the ILA in the efficacy of oxygenation and allowing circulatory support in the venoarterial mode. The isolated ILA thereby lost its role in lung transplantation. The PA/LA application may remain as one of the last indications.

The use in lung transplantation is now to bridge patients who are extubated with respiratory failure, to support patients in right heart failure, and also to be used during the transplant procedure and be continued thereafter.

Right heat failure requiring mechanical support is a different indication. The main role is to reestablish circulation rather than gas exchange. Therefore, venoarterial support is required. In most cases, partial flow is sufficient to relieve the symptoms of right heart failure, This procedure can be performed with the patient in an awake state using venoarterial ECMO with reduced flows.

Another potential use of ECMO in lung transplantation is during the lung transplant procedure. Different programs have developed, resulting in different opinions about the use of extracorporeal circulation in lung transplantation. When a program was derived from cardiac surgery, it seems natural to use cardiopulmonary bypass in every lung transplant procedure. An approach from thoracic surgeons is generally to do transplants without cardiopulmonary bypass and only call a cardiac surgeon when off-pump transplantation is not feasible. Venoarterial ECMO may be a suitable alternative to the heart-lung machine, especially when it needs to be continued after the transplant procedure.[25] Experience was generated when patients were bridged to transplantation on ECMO.[26] However, the anesthesia management of patients on ECMO is different from patients on conventional heart-lung machines, because meticulous hemostasis is required on ECMO and usually there is substantial concomitant cardiac blood flow. However, ECMO may reduce the cytokine response induced by the heart-lung machine. Because of these different approaches between major lung transplant programs, the use of ECMO in lung transplant procedures remains controversial.

Less controversial is the use of ECMO in severe primary graft dysfunction, because in some cases it represents the only potentially lifesaving alternative, so it should be available in all lung transplant centers. Some major centers prefer the use of venoarterial ECMO, because it reduces the pulmonary blood flow and thereby leads to reduction of lung edema and faster recovery of the graft.[27] Other centers prefer the use of venovenous cannulation,[28] because the overall complication rate is lower and it may be used for prolonged periods of time. Because there is no consensus in this regard, both methods may be used and similar overall outcomes.

An additional strategy for patients with pulmonary hypertension is the use of venoarterial ECMO as a bridge, during the transplantation, and for gradual weaning after transplantation according to the adaptation of the left heart as assessed by sequential evaluations by echocardiography.[29]

It is understandable from the history of extracorporeal gas exchange that, in the years when ECMO was associated with the most severe bleeding complications, neurologic insults, and cannulation problems, it was only indicated when all other measures failed. The new technologies allow a paradigm shift toward earlier indication and as an alternative to mechanical ventilation. It is the opinion of the author that these new principles are underserved and old decision making patterns still exist, leading to inferior results. Therefore, an overall trend for inferior outcomes is observed, leading to controversies about the use in bridging to transplantation.

FUTURE PERSPECTIVES

With the current improvements, ECMO therapy has matured and can be used in multiple configurations to support patients with respiratory and circulatory failure. The patterns of ECMO use from the time when ECMO technology evolved are still present. Bad experiences may lead to indications that are too late, leading to inferior outcomes.

The current technology allows the safe use of ECMO for a couple of weeks in venoarterial mode and several weeks in venovenous mode. Maturation of cannulation techniques has led to more percutaneous approaches and greater safety of operation, allowing operation of ECMO without a dedicated perfusionist present. Recent experience with extubated patients has led to a more modern approach and prolonged bridging times.[30]

However, the environment of an intensive care unit is still required and hospital discharge on ECMO is not advisable.

The status is comparable with extracorporeal ventricular assist devices, when patients were not allowed to leave the hospital.

What are the limiting factors? Modern oxygenators need to be exchanged within a couple of weeks. One main reason is that perfusion within the oxygenators is not homogeneous, leading to low-flow areas, where blood clotting is likely. In addition, the oxygenators need proper positioning and cannot be turned upside down.

In order to create a real artificial lung, more modifications to oxygenators are required, to allow for position changes, better geometry to extend lifetime, and also to reduce the requirement for anticoagulation. Reliable and automatic regulation of continuous gas flow is an additional essential issue. Cannulation techniques have evolved as a percutaneous approach to be used in the intensive care unit. However, durable long-term conduits still need to be designed.

However, many groups are working to increase the safety of the circuits to achieve an interim step called an ambulatory lung.[31]

With current oxygenator technologies, the development of full implantable systems is not feasible. To create an ambulatory artificial lung with extracorporeal components is necessary to allow patients to be discharged on such support systems. Such a system is needed for patients in lung failure who are not eligible for transplants.

When optimization of oxygenators, connection to reliable long-term pumps, regulated sweep gas flows, and suitable cannulae are developed and patients can be discharged, it will be possible to speak of a true artificial lung.

REFERENCES

1. Porepa LF, Starling RC. Destination therapy with left ventricular assist devices: for whom and when? Can J Cardiol 2014;30(3):296–303.
2. Hessel EA 2nd, Johnson DD, Ivey TD, et al. Membrane versus bubble oxygenator for cardiac operations. A prospective randomized study. J Thorac Cardiovasc Surg 1980;80(1):111–22.
3. Lim MW. History of extracorporeal oxygenation. Anaesthesia 2006;61:984–95.
4. Gibbon JH. An oxygenator with large surface area to Volume ratio. J Lab Clin Med 1939;24:1192–8.
5. Gibbon JH. Application of a mechanical heart and lung apparatus to cardiac surgery. Minn Med 1954;37:171–85.
6. Kirklin JW, Donald DE, Harshbarger HG, et al. Studies in extracorporeal circulation. I. Applicability of Gibbon-type pump-oxygenator to human intracardiac surgery: 40 cases. Ann Surg 1956;144(1): 2–8.
7. Ansell JE, Vandersalm T, Stephenson W, et al. In vivo survival of red blood cells processed by a bubble or membrane oxygenator during cardiopulmonary bypass surgery. Tex Heart Inst J 1986; 13(2):247–51.
8. Warren OJ, Smith AJ, Alexiou C, et al. The inflammatory response to cardiopulmonary bypass: part 1–mechanisms of pathogenesis. J Cardiothorac Vasc Anesth 2009;23(2):223–31.
9. Melrose DG, Bramson ML, Osborn JJ. Gerbode: the membrane oxygenator; some aspects of oxygen and carbon dioxide transport across polyethylene film. Lancet 1958;1(7029):1050–1.
10. Zapol WM, Snider MT, Hill JD, et al. Extracorporeal membrane oxygenation in severe acute respiratory failure. A randomized prospective study. JAMA 1979;242(20):2193–6.

11. Geelhoed GW, Adkins PC, Corso PJ, et al. Clinical effects of membrane lung support for acute respiratory failure. Ann Thorac Surg 1975;20(2):177–87.

12. Lewandowski K, Rossaint R, Pappert D, et al. High survival rate in 122 ARDS patients managed according to a clinical algorithm including extracorporeal membrane oxygenation. Intensive Care Med 1997; 23(8):819–35.

13. Kopp R, Dembinski R, Kuhlen R. Role of extracorporeal lung assist in the treatment of acute respiratory failure. Minerva Anestesiol 2006;72(6):587–95.

14. Morris AH, Wallace CJ, Menlove RL, et al. Randomized clinical trial of pressure-controlled inverse ratio ventilation and extracorporeal CO_2 removal for adult respiratory distress syndrome. Am J Respir Crit Care Med 1994;149(2 Pt 1):295–305.

15. Jurmann MJ, Haverich A, Demertzis S, et al. Extracorporeal membrane oxygenation as a bridge to lung transplantation. Eur J Cardiothorac Surg 1991;5(2):94–7.

16. Undar A, Wang S, Palanzo DA. Impact of polymethylpentene oxygenators on outcomes of all extracorporeal life support patients in the United States. Artif Organs 2013;37(12):1080–1.

17. Bein T, Weber F, Philipp A, et al. A new pumpless extracorporeal interventional lung assist in critical hypoxemia/hypercapnia. Crit Care Med 2006;34(5):1372–7.

18. Fischer S, Simon AR, Welte T, et al. Bridge to lung transplantation with the novel pumpless interventional lung assist device NovaLung. J Thorac Cardiovasc Surg 2006;131(3):719–23.

19. Zimmermann M, Bein T, Arlt M, et al. Pumpless extracorporeal interventional lung assist in patients with acute respiratory distress syndrome: a prospective pilot study. Crit Care 2009;13(1):R10.

20. Meyer AL, Strueber M, Tomaszek S, et al. Temporary cardiac support with a mini-circuit system consisting of a centrifugal pump and a membrane ventilator. Interact Cardiovasc Thorac Surg 2009;9(5):780–3.

21. Bein T, Zonies D, Philipp A, et al. Transportable extracorporeal lung support for rescue of severe respiratory failure in combat casualties. J Trauma Acute Care Surg 2012;73(6):1450–6.

22. Davies A, Jones D, Bailey M, et al. Extracorporeal membrane oxygenation for 2009 influenza A(H1N1) acute respiratory distress syndrome. JAMA 2009; 302(17):1888–95.

23. Gottlieb J, Warnecke G, Hadem J, et al. Outcome of critically ill lung transplant candidates on invasive respiratory support. Intensive Care Med 2012; 38(6):968–75.

24. Olsson KM, Simon A, Strueber M, et al. Extracorporeal membrane oxygenation in nonintubated patients as bridge to lung transplantation. Am J Transplant 2010;10(9):2173–8.

25. Bittner HB, Binner C, Lehmann S, et al. Replacing cardiopulmonary bypass with extracorporeal membrane oxygenation in lung transplantation operations. Eur J Cardiothorac Surg 2007;31(3):462–7.

26. Aigner C, Wisser W, Taghavi S, et al. Institutional experience with extracorporeal membrane oxygenation in lung transplantation. Eur J Cardiothorac Surg 2007;31(3):468–73.

27. Lang G, Aigner C, Winkler G, et al. Prolonged venoarterial extracorporeal membrane oxygenation after transplantation restores functional integrity of severely injured lung allografts and prevents the development of pulmonary graft failure in a pig model. J Thorac Cardiovasc Surg 2009;137(6): 1493–8.

28. Hartwig MG, Walczak R, Lin SS, et al. Improved survival but marginal allograft function in patients treated with extracorporeal membrane oxygenation after lung transplantation. Ann Thorac Surg 2012; 93(2):366–71.

29. Tudorache I, Sommer W, Kühn C, et al. Lung Transplantation for severe pulmonary hypertension-awake extracorporeal membrane oxygenation for postoperative left ventricular remodelling. Transplantation 2014. [Epub ahead of print].

30. Strueber M. Bridges to lung transplantation. Curr Opin Organ Transplant 2011;16(5):458–61.

31. Zhou X, Wang D, Sumpter R, et al. Long-term support with an ambulatory percutaneous paracorporeal artificial lung. J Heart Lung Transplant 2012; 31(6):648–54.

Index

Thorac Surg Clin 25 (2015) 115–119
http://dx.doi.org/10.1016/S1547-4127(14)00130-3
1547-4127/15/$ – see front matter © 2015 Elsevier Inc. All rights reserved.

thoracic.theclinics.com

Moving?

Make sure your subscription moves with you!

To notify us of your new address, find your **Clinics Account Number** (located on your mailing label above your name), and contact customer service at:

Email: journalscustomerservice-usa@elsevier.com

800-654-2452 (subscribers in the U.S. & Canada)
314-447-8871 (subscribers outside of the U.S. & Canada)

Fax number: 314-447-8029

Elsevier Health Sciences Division
Subscription Customer Service
3251 Riverport Lane
Maryland Heights, MO 63043

*To ensure uninterrupted delivery of your subscription, please notify us at least 4 weeks in advance of move.

Printed and bound by CPI Group (UK) Ltd, Croydon, CR0 4YY

03/10/2024

01040381-0009